Neonatal Hearing Screening

*The ultimate goal
of an infant hearing screening program
is to help the hearing-impaired child
achieve his or her full potential
through the timely provision
of medical, habilitative, and educational treatment.*

Laszlo K. Stein

Neonatal Hearing Screening

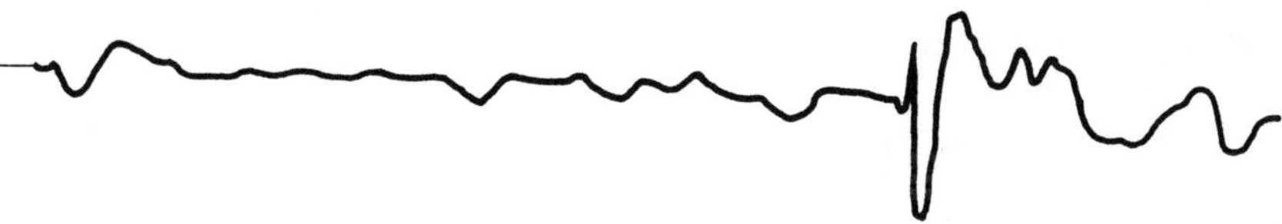

Edited by

Elca T. Swigart, Ph.D.

Speech and Hearing Center
The Reading Hospital and Medical Center
Reading, Pennsylvania

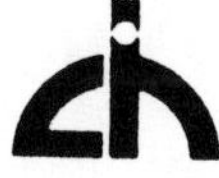

College-Hill Press, Inc., San Diego, California

College-Hill Press, Inc.
4284 1st Street
San Diego, CA 92105

Library of Congress Cataloging in Publication Data
Main entry under title:

Neonatal hearing screening.
   Includes index.
   1. Hearing disorders in children—Diagnosis.
2. Infants (Newborn)—Medical examination.
I. Swigart, Elca T., 1939-   . [DNLM: 1. Hearing
Disorders—diagnosis. 2. Hearing Tests—in infancy &
childhood. 3. Mass Screening—in infancy & children.
WV 271 N438]
RF291.5.C45N46 1986   618.92′0978   85-24289
ISBN 0-933014-18-X

Printed in the United States of America

To Vera Ruth Swigart

CONTENTS

Contributors ix

Preface xi

Acknowledgments xiii

Section I. **Information to Consider in Implementing a Neonatal Hearing Screening Program** 1

Chapter 1 The Rationale for Neonatal Hearing Screening 3
Marion P. Downs

Chapter 2 Screening Principles and Test Selection 21
Thomas J. Fria

Chapter 3 The Development and Outcome of the High-Risk Register 31
Katherine Pike Gerkin

Chapter 4 The Crib-o-gram in Neonatal Hearing Screening 47
George R. Marcellino

Chapter 5 The Auditory Brainstem Response in Neonatal Hearing Screening 67
John T. Jacobson and Martyn L. Hyde

Chapter 6 Follow-up of Infants in a Neonatal Hearing Screening Program 99
Laszlo K. Stein

Chapter 7 Considerations in the Implementation of a Hospital-Based Neonatal Hearing Screening Program 107
Elca T. Swigart

Chapter 8 Large-Scale High-Risk Neonatal Hearing Screening 123
Thomas M. Mahoney

Section II   **Model Programs**   **143**
Chapter 9   Model Program I: The Crib-o-gram   145
                    Adeline Clingan McClatchie and
                    Danielle M. Mikulich
Chapter 10   Model Program II: A High-Risk Register
                  and Auditory Brainstem Response   157
                    Kathi E. Kurmin and Thomas J. Fria
Chapter 11   Model Program III: A High-Risk Register,
                  Behavior Observation Audiometry, and
                  Auditory Brainstem Response   165
                    Wynnette J. Moneka
Chapter 12   Model Program IV: A High-Risk Register,
                  Crib-o-gram, and Auditory Brainstem
                  Response   183
                    Elca T. Swigart
Chapter 13   Model Program V: A High-Risk Register by
                  Computerized Search of Birth Certificates   223
                    Thomas M. Mahoney and
                    John G. Eichwald
Chapter 14   Model Program VI: An Infant Hearing
                  Assessment Foundation *SYNAP* Program   241
                    Alan Salamy and Christina Weyland

Author Index   **259**

Subject Index   **265**

CONTRIBUTORS

Marion P. Downs, M.S., D.H.S.
Audiology Division
University of Colorado Health
  Sciences Center
Denver, CO 80262

John G. Eichwald, M.A.
Bureau of Communicative
  Disorders
Utah Department of Health
Salt Lake City, UT 84113

Thomas J. Fria, Ph.D.
Audiology Division
Children's Hospital of Pittsburgh
Pittsburgh, PA 15213

Katherine Pike Gerkin, M.A.
Audiology Division
University of Colorado Health
  Sciences Center
Denver, CO 80262

Martyn L. Hyde, Ph.D.
Silverman Research Center
Mount Sinai Hospital
Toronto, Ontario M5G 1X5
Canada

John T. Jacobson, Ph.D.
Department of Communicative
  Disorders
University of Mississippi
University, MS 38677

Kathi E. Kurmin, M.S.
Audiology Division
Children's Hospital of Pittsburgh
Pittsburgh, PA 15213

Thomas M. Mahoney, Ph.D.
Bureau of Communicative
  Disorders
Utah Department of Health
Salt Lake City, UT 84113

George R. Marcellino, Ph.D.
Laserscope
Santa Clara, CA 95051

**Adeline Clingan McClatchie,
  L.C.S.T., Dip. Aud.**
Center for Children's
  Communication Disorders
Children's Hospital
Oakland, CA 94609

Danielle M. Mikulich, M.A.
Center for Children's
  Communication Disorders
Children's Hospital
Oakland, CA 94609

Wynnette J. Moneka, M.A.
Speech and Hearing Department
Christ Hospital
Oak Lawn, IL 60453

Alan Salamy, Ph.D.
Brain Behavior Research
  Center
University of California,
  San Francisco
Eldridge, CA 94531

Laszlo K. Stein, Ph.D.
Siegel Institute
Michael Reese Medical Center
Department of Surgery
  (Otolaryngology)
University of Chicago
Chicago, IL 60616

Elca T. Swigart, Ph.D.
Speech and Hearing Center
The Reading Hospital and
  Medical Center
Reading, PA 19603

Christina Weyland, M.A.
Department of Audiology
  and Speech Pathology
Methodist Hospital
Indianapolis, IN 46202

PREFACE

The importance of early identification and habilitation of children with hearing impairment has been recognized, and efforts are being made to detect hearing loss as early as possible. A rather recent evolution in early identification is the screening of infants shortly after birth. Although the value of hearing screening is almost universally accepted, the determination of the most suitable screening method for neonates has not been fully resolved.

The contributors to this text have a significant amount of clinical experience in dealing with the identification of hearing loss in the infant population. The editor has not attempted to reconcile differences of views. The aim of this book is to present a broad coverage of information emanating from diverse sources in the emergent area of hearing screening.

This text is intended as a guide for the professional who is interested in implementing a neonatal hearing screening program. It is designed to assist the audiologist, neonatologist, pediatrician, otolaryngologist, nurse, or hospital administrator in soliciting interprofessional cooperation in the development of an efficient and cost-effective program. Those professionals who are willing to accept the challenge and rewards of neonatal hearing screening must recognize the strengths and limitations involved in current screening procedures. They must also realize the importance of the totality of the screening program, which should encompass not only the initial identification, but also the follow-up diagnostic testing and the eventual habilitation of the hearing-impaired child.

The text is divided into two sections. The chapters in the first section are constructed to provide the reader with information to consider in implementing a hearing screening program. Suggestions for weighing the alternatives and making a sound decision concerning the screening method that best fulfills the requirements of the intended program are provided. Guidance concerning actual implementation of a screening program and establishment of necessary follow-up procedures is also offered. The second section details protocols of model programs and illustrates the diversity of settings in which various hearing screening methods and follow-up diagnostic testing can be incorporated.

It is hoped that this text will be viewed as a reference and not as a standard that is inflexible. The information is intended to be adapted to many situations, taking into account the resources of the institutions and localities. Variations and innovations that improve neonatal hearing screening are encouraged. The importance of searching for better techniques to provide more efficient identification of hearing loss early in life cannot be overemphasized. To make progress tomorrow, we must strive to improve on the knowledge and techniques available today.

ACKNOWLEDGMENTS

I wish to express my sincere appreciation to the contributors for their enthusiasm and cooperation and for the sophistication they have brought to this text. A special thank you is extended to my secretary, Grace Heist, and my editorial consultants and proofreaders, Betsy Hirsch Katz and Barbara Nusbaum Andrew. I would like to acknowledge the support of the administration of The Reading Hospital and Medical Center during this endeavor. Marion Downs deserves special credit for continued encouragement throughout my years of interest in neonatal hearing screening. Finally, to family, friends, and co-workers, thank you for your patience and understanding.

SECTION I

INFORMATION TO CONSIDER IN IMPLEMENTING A NEONATAL HEARING SCREENING PROGRAM

Chapter 1

The Rationale for Neonatal Hearing Screening

Marion P. Downs

Hearing impairment is considered second only to arthritis as the most prevalent chronic disease in the United States. Yet the demographic figures on hearing loss are hard to pin down. They are dependent on two factors: the degree of loss and the age of occurrence of the loss. Application of prevalence rates for severely and profoundly deafened individuals reports by Schein and Delk (1974) to the 1984 population of the United States (233,981,000) produces the following projected rates:

Degree of Loss	Age of Onset	Number	Rate/100,000
Deaf	All ages	2,042,654	873
	Prevocational	474,981	203
	Prelingual	233,981	100

The prelingually deaf are the purview of this book, and the incidence figure of 1 in 1000 is acceptable for those with severe and profound losses at birth. But ever since newborn screening programs have been in operation, most are finding that the incidence of those born with mild to profound degrees of permanent hearing impairment is at least 1 in 750, as more mildly impaired children are included in the statistics.

When this figure is applied to the 3,600,000 births per year in the United States, it means that 4800 hearing impaired infants will be born yearly, bringing to 360,000 the over-all number of prelingual, or congenital deaf in the United States.

The figures are markedly different when all degrees of hearing loss and all ages are considered (Schein and Delk, 1974):

Degree of Loss	Age of Onset	Number	Rate/100,000
All hearing impaired	All ages	15,449,765	6,603
Significant bilateral	All ages	2,042,654	873

The numbers given here for all hearing impaired do not take into consideration new data on the extent of chronic, recurrent ear disease—chiefly middle ear effusion (MEE)—in young children. This disease results in hearing losses of 26 to 31 dB average (McDermott, Giebink, Le, Harford, and Paparella, 1983), which is a significant loss for young children during their early language-learning years. Thirty-three percent of all children will have had three or more attacks of MEE by 3 years of age (Teele, Klein, and Rosner, 1984). Using these statistics, the following figures will apply for the United States population in 1984:

Degree of Loss	Age of Onset	Number aged 3 years or less	Rate/ 100,000
Mild conductive	Birth to 3 years	3,621,000	33,000

The high incidence of MEE has prompted the Academy of Pediatrics to issue a policy statement recommending that children who have had consistent or recurrent MEE for 3 months must have an audiological assessment and a communication evaluation.

Although the figures on MEE may not seem relevant to newborn hearing screening, it is known that in the main targeted nurseries for newborn screening—the intensive care units—as many as 30 to 35 percent of those infants will have acute suppurative otitis media (Berman, Balkany, and Simmons, 1978; McDonald, 1967) and will be identified in some screening programs as hearing impaired. This number increases rapidly in the first 6 months of life.

All these figures are important to the justification of expenditures for newborn hearing screening programs. How much could society save if all prelingually deaf children were identified at birth and given habilitation that would allow them to develop the language skills and the earning capacities of those who were deafened after language had been learned? According to Schein and Delk (1974), the prelingually deaf earn 18 percent less than the postlingually deaf. Translated into economic figures, many billions of dollars would be added to the over-all United States economy yearly if the congenitally deaf could be identified at birth and habilitated.

In addition to manpower earnings, one must take into consideration the costs of education and therapy for the hearing impaired—costs that could markedly be reduced by early identification and habilitation. Children identified and given early educational management could be mainstreamed into regular school programs throughout their school life or mainstreamed earlier than would have otherwise been possible, reducing the costs of special training. Figures extrapolated from 1969 data collected by the U.S. Department of Health, Education, and Welfare (1968) and applied to the present population indicate that special education, resource services, and speech-language-hearing therapy and training for education is approximately $500,000,000 per year. Easily half of that expense could be saved if hearing-impaired children could arrive at school age ready to be mainstreamed.

Such amounts easily justify the expenditures necessary to identify hearing losses at birth, especially when one adds the improved quality of life that results from such early identification. For those people, the joy of being able to communicate more adequately with family, friends, and peers is worth any price. The deepest concern of professionals, legislators, and the general public should be directed toward this major problem.

THE HANDICAP OF DEAFNESS

The 18 percent differential between the earning power of the deaf population and that of the general population represents the degree of language dysfunction that results when hearing losses are not detected until after critical periods of language development have passed. Although the language level of the deaf may be said to be grossly proportional to the degree of loss, an even greater influence is the age at which the loss was identified and habilitation begun. Given similar degrees of loss, the earlier the identification is made, the better the language skill (Greenstein et al., 1976).

Some crucial developmental patterns in the language skills of the hearing impaired illustrate these points. A number of reports have been made indicating that the language level of deaf students improves slowly in the first three grades and then levels off at the fourth grade to a permanent fourth grade equivalent level. Table 1–1 shows the slow progression of grade equivalent language scores as reported by a Gallaudet College survey in 1971 (Reis, 1973). A significant fact is that at age 6 years, the language level of the deaf children is at age level or better, but from that time on, it fails to improve at a parallel rate with grade levels. The inexorable toll of the lack of lan-

Table 1–1. Plateauing of Scores of Paragraph Meaning Subtests of the Stanford Achievement Test on Students in Schools for the Deaf and Hard-of-Hearing

Age	Grade Equivalent Scores
6	1.96
10	2.24
16	3.85
19	4.36
20	4.23

From P. Reis (1973). Academic achievement test; results of a national testing program for impaired students. Office of Demographic Studies, Gallaudet College, Washington, DC.

guage experience during early critical periods is seen. The fact is that perhaps very few of the children in the Gallaudet study had been identified as hearing impaired before the age of 3 years, because at that time, the best average age of identification was 2.7 years (Bergstrom, Hemenway, and Downs, 1971).

The Gallaudet report involved mainly deaf and severely hard-of-hearing students in special schools or classrooms in the United States. Another, more recent report covered all hearing-impaired children in the Iowa public schools (Davis, Shepard, Stelmachowitz, and Gorga, 1981). It showed a similar trend toward a plateauing or regression in the amount of improvement in language measures made by these children as they grew older. Table 1–2 illustrates the regression. The relevant fact in this study is that of the 1250 children covered in the study, only 29 had been identified as hearing-impaired before the age of 3 years.

CRITICAL LEARNING PERIODS

It is probably simplistic to say that all the language deficits illustrated in these reports were caused by failure to identify and remediate the hearing losses at an appropriate time, but a large body of knowledge exists regarding the importance of instituting remedial measures at a very early stage in the child's life if he is to achieve his potential for language learning. The data are difficult to ignore when the regression shown above is considered.

The reasons for this regression were recognized as early as 1966 when two prominent linguistics (Chomsky, 1966; Lenneberg, 1967) propounded their theories that language is an innate function, time-locked to early periods of development when the brain is at its most plastic state and can implement the language input it receives into the highest language cognition. The periods that have been sug-

Table 1–2. Language Age Versus Chronological Age in Hearing-Impaired Students, Iowa

Age Range	Language Skills
H/L Av. 50–80 dB; 500 Hz $\leqslant$ 50 dB H/L	
5–8 years	$\leqslant$ 1 year below normal
8–11 years	$\geqslant$ 3 years below normal
>12 years	$\geqslant$ 5 years below normal
H/L Av. 25–50 dB; 500 Hz $\leqslant$ 30 dB	
5–8 years	1 year below normal
8–11 years	2.5 years below normal
H/L Av. 25–50 dB; 500 Hz >30 dB	
5–8 years	1 year below normal
8–11 years	2.8 years below normal
H/L Av. >80 dB	
5–8 years	2.3 years below normal
8–11 years	3 years below normal
>12 years	6.5 years below normal

Information to compile this table from J. M. Davis, N. T. Shepard, P. G. Stelmachowitz, and M. P. Gorga (1981). Characteristics of hearing-impaired children in the public schools: Part II—Psychoeducational data. *Journal of Speech and Hearing Disorders,* *46,* (2), 130–137.

gested as critical to this function range from birth to 3 years. Ruben and Rapin (1980) have described the evidence for an anatomical basis for an early plasticity of the brain, requiring stimulation in the first 3 years of life if auditory perceptions and language learning are to be implemented:

> Available information would indicate that the maturation of the auditory system is centripetal, proceeding from the inner ear to the auditory cortex. Environmental sound would appear to have its greatest effect in shaping auditory ability from the time the inner ear and eighth nerve first become functional to the time when maturation of the central nervous system is achieved.

This maturation is perhaps complete by 3 years of age, according to Webster and Webster's (1980) extrapolation from animal studies. Inasmuch as language is a biological function, it, too, is subject to the same constraints of early plasticity as the auditory system.

Confirmatory evidence for the importance of early implementation of language learning has come from many sources. Even in the case of normal hearing children, early intervention for children who might be impoverished by their environment has been shown to be effective. Guinagh and Jester (1981) reviewed all the early intervention programs reported in the United States. They found that those children in programs that involve early infant home language stimulation programs showed measurably greater long-term gains when compared with children who received later interventions or who did not receive intervention. Table 1–3 shows an analysis of these programs.

Additional information comes from a consortium on longitudinal studies (Schweinhart and Weikart, 1980), reporting that the intervention programs that showed the longest duration of gains were those starting at birth and involving the parents. "The earlier the better" seems to be the consensus.

Although few controlled studies have been made on the hearing-impaired population that demonstrate plasticity, a group of researchers at Lexington School for the Deaf carried out the most definitive study (Greenstein et al., 1976). They compared children who had been admitted to the school before 16 months of age with another group that had been admitted between 16 and 24 months of age. A battery of language and speech tests were given over a period ending when the children were 40 months of age, and an informal measure of mother-infant communication was made. The results showed that the children admitted prior to 16 months of age were consistently superior to those admitted later in all aspects and at all age levels through 40 months. The learning abilities of the children were clearly related to the time remediation was begun. It is clear that there is no substitute for identification at birth.

THE NEED FOR NEONATAL HEARING SCREENING

Despite knowledge of the advantage of early habilitation for hearing loss, there has not been satisfactory movement toward neonatal identification. In 1971, Bergstrom and associates reported that parents of deaf children suspected the hearing losses when children were an average of 11 months of age; they told their physicians of the concern at this time. But the children were an average of 27 months before the losses were finally remediated. In 1984, Bergstrom again made a survey, this time in California, and it showed no improvement in the age of beginning remediation—the children were still 27 months before their problems were finally brought to habilitation. Contrast this study with those that show the average time of remediation to be 3 months in a neonatal screening program using the risk register and ABR testing (Gerkin, 1984).

Other alternatives to neonatal screening have been proposed. W. Frankenburg (personal communication, 1981) believes that physicians should be responsible for screening hearing of infants at well-baby visits. But as Bergstrom's figures show, there has been no

Table 1–3. I. Q. and School Advantages Produced by Early Intervention Versus that of Non-Intervention

Program	Beginning Age	Final Eval. Age	I. Q. Interv. Group	I. Q. Control Group	No. in Spec. Ed. Classes (%)	
					Interv.	Contr.
Gordon	3 mo.	10.3 yr.	88.1	77.8	9.1	29.2
Levenstein	2 yr.	9 yr.	101.9	93.6	13.7	39.1

From B. J. Guinagh and R. E. Jester (1981). Long-term effects of infant stimulation programs. *Advances in Behavioral Pediatrics, 2,* 81–110. Copyright 1981 by JAI Press. Reprinted by permission.

movement in that direction in the past 14 years. Another alternative is screening at well-baby public health clinics—an option that has been demonstrated to be effective in Israel (Feinmesser and Tell, 1976), Sweden (Stensland-Junker, 1974), Poland (Borkowska-Gaertig et al., 1974) and other countries. These are all countries with social-ized medicine, where 80 to 90 percent of all children receive their health care at the public clinics. In the United States, the majority of children are managed by private physicians, so public clinic screening would not be as effective here.

Unfortunately, the only time prior to school age when the entire population is available for testing in the United States is in the new-born nursery. Therefore, we must adapt our programs to our own conditions and use the newborn nursery for hearing screening.

What Is Screening?

A customary definition of screening is "a process of applying to large numbers of individuals certain rapid, simple measures that will identify those individuals with high probability of disorders in the function tested" (Northern and Downs, 1984).

All screening programs in the public health domain are subject to the following criteria, which have been enunciated by public health officials (Frankenburg, 1970; North, 1975):

1. Occurrence of the disease frequent enough to warrant mass screening.
2. Amenability of the disease to treatment or prevention that will change the expected outcome.
3. Availability of facilities for diagnosis and treatment.
4. Cost of screening reasonably commensurate with benefits to the individual.
5. Acceptance by the public and the professional community.
6. A screening tool that validly differentiates the disease from non-disease.

Neonatal screening programs are able to meet all these criteria, but the last criterion must be constantly reevaluated whenever a new screening tool is introduced. This criterion is of extreme importance and should be examined further.

The validity of any screening test for hearing is determined first by the agreement between the rating of a child as positive (abnormal) on the screening test and his rating as positive on the diagnostic threshold test, and second by the agreement between the screening test's classification of a child as negative (normal) and the threshold diagnostic test's designation of him as normal. The accuracy of a screening test in correctly identifying the positive (abnormal) subjects is called *sensitivity;* its accuracy in classifying correctly the negative (normal) subjects is called *specificity.* Table 1-4 describes the formulation of sensitivity and specificity.

All neonatal hearing screening tools should be subjected to an analysis of sensitivity and specificity. However, to do so would require that an entire newborn population be followed up with extensive diagnostic tests. Inasmuch as that would not be economically feasible for large populations, most studies apply the validation test only to the cases that were abnormal according to the screening. This leaves the normal cases untested by the validation tool. Consequently, this approach cannot truly demonstrate the validity of the tool. There has been a more recent trend to attempt to validate screening on smaller, select groups, such as intensive care unit graduates.

With the use of the ABR, the screening tool may also be the validation tool, so modern newborn screening programs may be unique in the screening field. However, if the high-risk register is considered as a screening tool in itself, it needs to be examined and revised continually in the light of sensitivity and specificity.

HISTORY OF NEONATAL HEARING SCREENING

Recognizing the need to identify congenital deafness at birth, in the 1950s a number of investigators throughout the world began to explore techniques for such screening. In Sweden, Wedenberg (1956) and Froding (1960) described using the auropalpebral response (APR) in response to sound as the technique of choice. This response was used and enlarged upon by Downs and and Sterritt (1964) in the United States, who described the APR, the startle response, and a variety of subtle head and limb movements as valid responses. The stimulus they developed was a 3000 Hz narrow band, chosen because it seemed appropriate to identify typical high-frequency sen-

Table 1–4. Calculation of Sensitivity and Specificity*

Screen Test	Diseased	Non-Diseased	
Positive	a	b	
Negative	c	d	
	a + c	b + d	a+b+c+d

*Sensitivity: Percent of diseased designated positive with screen test a/(a + c).
Specificity: Percent of nondiseased designated negative with screen test d/(b + d).
False positive = b; false negative = c.
Results are random if sensitivity = % positive a/(a + c) = (a + b) /
  (a + b + c + d).
Results are random if sensitivity + specificity = 100%.
Note: The same computations are made for co-positivity and co-negativity.

From J. Northern and M. Downs (1983). *Hearing in children (3rd ed.)* (p. 201). Copyright 1983 by Williams and Wilkins Co., Baltimore. Reprinted by permission.

sorineural losses. They demonstrated that those responses could be agreed upon by two independent observers.

Subsequently, Downs and Hemenway (1969) reported on using the responses in screening 17,000 newborns and identifying 9 deaf infants. As their program continued, however, it was noted that almost all the infants who were found to be deaf fell into some recognized categories of etiologies. Further, other reports questioned the sensitivity of a test using behavioral responses that rely on the subjective evaluation of observers (Ling, Ling, and Doehring, 1970; Goldstein and Tait, 1971).

In 1970, Downs approached the American Speech and Hearing Association with a request that a joint committee, composed of representatives from the Academy of Otolaryngology, the Academy of Pediatrics, and the American Speech and Hearing Association, be formed to evaluate the status of newborn screening. In 1971, this committee issued a statement that discouraged mass behavioral screening of newborns but urged further research. Shortly thereafter, the committee issued another statement recommending audiological testing of all newborns who fell into certain high-risk categories. The testing recommended was an ''in-depth audiological evaluation of hearing.'' Here again, a diagnostic procedure was incorporated into a screening program.

In the 1970s, there emerged two objective techniques for testing the hearing of newborns: Auditory Brainstem Response (ABR) audiometry and the Crib-o-gram (see Chapters 4 and 5 of this text). A revised statement of the Joint Committee in 1982 accommodated the new advancements by recommending that ''the initial screening should include the observation of behavioral or electrophysiologic response to sound.'' No specific device was recommended. The committee also revised the categories that were to be included in the high-risk register. The entire statement of the committee can be found in Appendix 1–A.

In establishing the high-risk categories, the committee was influenced by reports from Mencher (1974); McCulloch, Stick, and Mencher (1974); Cunningham (1970); and Feinmesser and Tell (1976). The latter study was the most extensive. It covered 17,731 newborns to whom a high-risk register was applied, and 23 deaf infants were eventually identified. Sixty-five percent of the deaf children had been on the high-risk register. It is interesting to note that 5 of the 23 hearing-impaired children had been cleared for hearing at 7 months of age and were later found at 3- to 4-year-old well-baby examinations to have losses. Thus, the losses appeared to be acquired and could not be expected to be identified by the Register, giving more credence to the register than the 65 percent figure would indicate.

The categories of risk selected by the joint committee are subject to change as medical advances continue. There may come a time when hyperbilirubinemia may no longer be a cause of deafness owing to the use of exchange transfusions and phototherapy. Rubella may all but disappear as a cause, because the rubella vaccination is reducing the number of cases in the population. What may take their place in prevalence is cytomegalovirus (CMV) and hypoxia. CMV has escalated as a cause of deafness, constituting 40 percent of all deafness found in a large study in Sweden (Harris, Ahlfors, Ivarsson, Lernmark, and Svanberg, 1984). Because more children are being kept alive by advanced techniques in intensive care nurseries, hypoxia and low birth rate may also rise to alarming proportions as causes of deafness in the future.

At the time of issuance of the 1982 statement of the joint committee, a representative of the American Nurses Association had been added to the committee roster, but, by 1984, this group withdrew its representation due to the travel costs involved. As presently constituted, the Committee consists of two representatives from the three original associations. The American Speech-Language-Hearing Association has now formed its own standing committee on infant hearing, which will make recommendations to its representatives on the Joint Committee.

REVISED DEFINITION OF SCREENING

The definition of screening described heretofore must be revised in view of the uniqueness of current neonatal screening constraints, because neonatal screening deviates in important ways from that definition. As presently practiced, many neonatal screening programs use ABR testing as the screening tool. ABR is not a "rapid, simple measure" as specified in the earlier definition; rather, it is an extremely powerful diagnostic tool and, in that respect, does not fit the definition. It seems necessary to construct an individualized definition for this new type of screening program—one that takes into consideration the uniqueness of this new approach to screening.

Traditionally, hearing screening procedures use one stimulus intensity that is not a threshold level and require a "yes" or "no" answer, indicating whether or not the listener heard it. With ABR testing, however, many practitioners develop a rich variety of threshold or near-threshold information, plus suprathreshold information, that can in reality be termed *diagnostic data*. The ABR instrument is thus a diagnostic tool used as a nominal "screening tool"; in actual fact, ABR is the criterion test of hearing in the neonatal population. So the classic definition of screening does not fit this condition.

In addition, at the present time, some of the electrophysiological tests used for screening are being done on a pre-selected population of newborn infants, selected by applying to the entire newborn population the procedure of the high-risk register. The register itself meets the definition of screening in that it does screen out those children who have a "high probability of disorders in the function tested," but it is not the actual test instrument. Even when the register is used to identify infants who will then be referred for behavioral audiological evaluation rather than ABR (as in some programs), that behavioral audiologic evaluation is not a screening procedure, because it is done by a professional person under diagnostic conditions.

A new definition of neonatal hearing screening that incorporates the new conditions may be "A process that identifies from the newborn population a small group of infants with a high probability of hearing impairment who are then given diagnostic hearing tests." This definition more accurately describes many programs currently in operation.

CONCLUSIONS

At the present time, we know how to identify hearing losses in infants, we know when to identify them, and we have sophisticated tools and techniques at our command to do so. Yet it is possible that fewer than 5 percent of the newborn population in this country is being tested with screening procedures. The reasons seem obscure.

Expense may not be the answer, because a program using the high-risk register with audiological follow-up can be an inexpensive procedure. The states of Colorado (Weber, personal communication, 1985) and Utah (Chapter 13) are carrying on effective programs using that procedure; the province of Manitoba in Canada is also currently implementing a province-wide cost-effective program (Magian, 1981). It does not seem to be a matter of legislation, because some of the states conducting programs have no laws making neonatal screening mandatory. By a strange quirk, some of the states that do have legislation mandating newborn screening appear to have less effective screening that those without such laws.

The critical feature that separates effective from ineffective programs seems to be the strategy that is used to identify the high-risk population. Those states using the Birth Record to compile most of the risk categories appear to be effective, but also effective are various hospital programs, some of which use volunteers in setting up the high-risk register. Each locality has to adapt the program to its particular situation.

In hospitals, one stumbling block to implementing hearing screening programs (especially those using ABR) has been the assumption of the responsibility for the neonatal screening by a variety of departments. A total identification program should be managed by a person with training in acoustics, psychoacoustics, hearing rehabilitation, audiology, audiometry, and auditory physiology, as well as the electronic skills specific to the ABR instrument. Such a person can follow up with behavioral tests and can implement the habilitation program for identified children. Such a person is also the appropriate one to interpret the ABR results. Until people with this type of training become the managers of the entire project, neonatal programs cannot become the comprehensive whole they should be. Although an interdisciplinary approach is needed for diagnosis and habilitation, a splintering off of the screening program with ''responsibility'' divided between disciplines is not in the best interests of the hearing-impaired infant.

For the future, the ideal neonatal screening program would be one that tests every baby in the newborn nurseries, because the high-risk register will always have reduced sensitivity despite all the efforts to make it more inclusive of all etiologies. Such testing of the entire newborn population is the face of the future for neonatal hearing screening. With continued technological improvements, it may soon be a reality.

The chapters in this book explain the current state of the art of neonatal hearing screening.

REFERENCES

Bergstrom, L., Hemenway, W. G., and Downs, M. P. (1971). A High Risk Registry to find congenital deafness. *Otolaryngology Clinics of North America, 4,* 369–399.

Bergstrom, L. (1984, March). *Congenital deafness.* Paper presented at the Colorado Otology–Audiology Workshop, Aspen, CO.

Berman, S. A., Balkany, T. J., and Simmons, M. A. (1978). Otitis media in the neonatal intensive care unit. *Pediatrics, 62,* 198–202.

Borkowska-Gaertig, D., Urbanska, I., Sobieszanska-Radoszewska, L., Rzedowskaz, and Rola-Janicki, A. (1974). Evaluation of the three-stage hearing testing programme for children in Poland. In G. Mencher (Ed.), *Early identification of hearing loss.* Basel: S. Karger.

Chomsky, N. (1966). *Aspects of the theory of syntax.* Cambridge, MA: MIT Press.

Cunningham, G. C. (1970). *Earlier recognition of handicapping conditions in childhood. Proceedings of a Bi-Regional Institute.* University of California, Berkeley: School of Public Health.

Davis, J. M., Shepard, N. T., Stelmachowitz, P. G., and Gorga, M. P. (1981). Characteristics of hearing-impaired children in the public schools: Part II—Psychoeducational data. *Journal of Speech and Hearing Disorders, 46,* 130–137.

Downs, M. P., and Sterritt, G. M. (1964). Identification audiometry for neonates. A preliminary report. *Journal of Auditory Research, 4,* 69–80.

Downs, M. P., and Hemenway, W. G. (1969). Report on the hearing screening of 17,000 neonates. *International Audiology, 8,* 72–76.

Feinmesser, M., and Tell, L. (1976). Evaluation of methods for detecting hearing impairment in infancy and early childhood. In G. T. Mencher (Ed.), *Early identification of hearing loss* (pp. 102–113). Basel: S. Karger.

Frankenburg, W. (1970). Evaluation of screening procedures. In E. M. Gold (Ed.), *Earlier recognition of handicapping conditions in childhood: Proceedings of a bi-regional institute* (pp. 42–51). University of California, Berkeley: School of Public Health.

Froding, C. A. (1960). Acoustic investigation of newborn infants. *Acta Otolaryngologica, 52,* 31–41.

Gerkin, K. (1984). The high risk register for deafness: A tutorial. *ASHA, 26* (3), 17–23.

Goldstein, R., and Tait, C. (1971). Critique of neonatal hearing evaluation. *Journal of Speech and Hearing Disorders, 36,* 3–18.

Greenstein, J. M., Greenstein, B. B., McConville, K., et al. (1976). *Mother-infant communication and language acquisition in deaf infants.* New York: Lexington School for the Deaf.

Guinagh, B. J., and Jester, R. E. (1981). Long-term effects of infant stimulation programs. *Advances in Behavioral Pediatrics, 2,* 81–110.

Harris, S., Ahlfors, K., Ivarsson, S., Lernmark, B., and Svanberg, L. (1984). Congenital cytomegalovirus infection and sensorineural hearing loss. *Ear and Hearing, 5,* 352–355.

Lenneberg, E. H. (1967). *Biological foundations of language.* New York: John Wiley and Sons.

Ling, D., Ling, A. H., and Doehring, D. G. (1970). Stimulus response and observer variables in the auditory screening of newborn infants. *Journal of Speech and Hearing Research, 13,* 9–18.

Magian, V.deC. (1981). The risk register for infant deafness as implemented in Manitoba. *Canadian Journal of Public Health, 72,* 181–185.

McCulloch, B. J., Stick, S. L., and Mencher, G. T. (1974). The University of Nebraska neonatal hearing project—One year later. In G. Mencher (Ed.), *Early identification of hearing loss.* Basel: S. Karger.

McDermott, J. C., Giebink, G. S., Le, C. T., Harford, E. R. and Paparella, M. M. (1983). Children with persistent otitis media. *Archives of Otolaryngology, 109,* 360–362.

McDonald, A. (1967). Children of very low birthweight. *MEIV Research Monograph No. 1.* London: Heinemann.

Mencher, G. T. (1974). A program for neonatal hearing screening. *Audiology, 13,* 495–500.

North, F. A. (1975). Urinalysis. In W. K. Frankenburg and B. W. Camp (Eds.), *Pediatric screening tests* (pp. 239–252). Springfield, IL: Charles C Thomas.

Northern, J., and Downs, M. (1984). *Hearing in children* (3rd ed.). Baltimore: Williams and Wilkins.

Reis, P. (1973). *Academic achievement test: Results of a national testing program for impaired students.* Office of Demographic Studies, Gallaudet College, Washington, DC.

Ruben, R. J., and Rapin, I. (1980). Plasticity of the developing auditory system. *Annals of Otology, Rhinology, Laryngology, 89,* 303–311.

Schein, J. D., and Delk, M. T. (1974). *The deaf population of the United States.* Silver Spring, MD: National Association of the Deaf.

Schweinhart, L. J., and Weikart, D. P. (1980). Young children grow up: The effects of the Perry Preschool Program on youths through age 15. *Monographs of the High/Scope Educational Research Foundation* (No. 7). Ypsilanti, MI: The High Scope Press.

Stensland-Junker, K. (1974). BOEL—A child welfare program for early screening of communication abilities. In G. Mencher (Ed.), *Early identification of hearing loss.* Basel: S. Karger.

Teele, D. W., Klein, J. O., Rosner, B. A., and The Greater Boston Otitis Media Study Group (1984). Otitis media with effusion during the first three years of life and development of speech and language. *Pediatrics, 74,* 282–287.

U.S. Department H.E.W., N.I.H., P.H.S. (1968). *Human Communication and Its Disorders—An Overview.* A report by the sub-committee on human communications and its disorders, Grant No. NB 07612.

Webster, D. B., and Webster, M. (1980). Mouse brainstem auditory nuclei development. *Annals of Otology, Rhinology, and Laryngology* (Suppl. 89), *68,* 254–256.

Wedenberg, E. (1956). Auditory tests on newborn infants. *Acta Otolaryngologica, 46,* 446–461.

Appendix **1-A**

Joint Committee on Infant Hearing Position Statement

Early detection of hearing impairment in the affected infant is important for medical treatment and subsequent educational intervention to ensure development of communication skills.

In 1973, the Joint Committee on Infant Hearing Screening recommended identifying infants at risk for hearing impairment by means of five criteria and suggested follow-up audiological evaluation of these infants until accurate assessments of hearing could be made. Since the incidence of moderate to profound hearing loss in the at-risk infant group is 2.5% to 5%, audiologic testing of this group is warranted. Acoustic testing of all newborn infants has a high incidence of false-positive and false-negative results and is not universally recommended.

Recent research suggests the need for expansion and clarification of the 1973 criteria. This 1982 statement expands the risk criteria and makes recommendations for the evaluation and treatment of the hearing-impaired infant.

I. IDENTIFICATION

A. Risk Criteria

The factors that identify those infants who are AT RISK for having hearing impairment include the following:

1. A family history of childhood hearing impairment.
2. Congenital perinatal infection (e.g., cytomegalovirus, rubella, herpes, toxoplasmosis, syphilis).

3. Anatomic malformations involving the head or neck (e.g., dysmorphic appearance, including syndromal and nonsyndromal abnormalities, overt or submucous cleft palate, morphologic abnormalities of the pinna).
4. Birthweight less than 1500 gm.
5. Hyperbilirubinemia at level exceeding indications for exchange transfusion.
6. Bacterial meningitis, especially from *H. influenzae*.
7. Severe asphyxia, which may include infants with Apgar scores of 0–3 who fail to institute spontaneous respiration by 10 minutes and those with hypotonia persisting to 2 hours of age.

B. Screening Procedures

The hearing of infants who manifest any item on the list of risk criteria should be screened, preferably under supervision of an audiologist, optimally by 3 months of age, but not later than 6 months of age. The initial screening should include the observation of behavioral or electrophysiological response to sound.* If consistent electrophysiological or behavioral responses are detected at appropriate sound levels, the screening process will be considered complete except in those cases in which there is a probability of a progressive hearing loss (e.g., family history of delayed onset, degenerative disease, intra-uterine infections). If results of an initial screening of an infant manifesting any risk criteria are equivocal, the infant should be referred for diagnostic testing.

II. DIAGNOSIS FOR INFANTS FAILING SCREENING

A. Diagnostic evaluation of an infant under 6 months of age includes:
1. General physical examination and history including:
   a. Examination of the head and neck
   b. Otoscopy and otomicroscopy
   c. Identification of relevant physical abnormalities
   d. Laboratory tests such as urinalysis and diagnostic tests for perinatal infections

---

*This Committee has no recommendations at this time regarding any specific device.

From Position Statement by Joint Committee on Infant Hearing, 1982, *ASHA*, 24(12), pp. 1017–1018. Copyright 1982 by American Speech-Language-Hearing Association. Reprinted by permission.

    2. Comprehensive audiological evaluation:
      a. Behavioral history
      b. Behavioral observation audiometry
      c. Testing of auditory evoked potentials, if indicated.
B. After the age of 6 months, the following are also recommended:
    1. Communication skills evaluation
    2. Acoustic immitance measurements
    3. Selected tests of development

III. MANAGEMENT OF THE HEARING-IMPAIRED INFANT

Habilitation of the hearing-impaired infant may begin while the diagnostic evaluation is in process. The Committee recommends, however, that whenever possible, the diagnostic process should be completed and habilitation begun by the age of 6 months. Services to the hearing-impaired infant under 6 months of age include:

A. Medical Management
    1. Reevaluation
    2. Treatment
    3. Genetic evaluation and counseling when indicated
B. Audiologic Management
    1. Ongoing audiological assessment
    2. Selection of hearing aid(s)
    3. Family counseling
C. Psychoeducational Management
    1. Formulation of an individualized educational plan
    2. Information about the implications of hearing impairment

After the age of 6 months, the hearing-impaired infant becomes easier to manage in a habilitation plan but he or she will require the services listed above.

Chapter **2**

Screening Principles and Test Selection*

Thomas J. Fria

Informative discussions of the principles of screening and the characteristics of tests are not commonly found in the audiologic literature. Much of the material that follows was adapted from a paper by Thorner and Remein (1982) and a chapter that appeared in a text by Northern and Downs (1974).

The main objective of screening is to rule out disease or impairment in a population that consists of both impaired and unimpaired individuals. This can be done in a number of ways. For example, generating a list or register of newborns who present with one of the high-risk factors for congenital hearing loss is a form of screening, because babies who appear on the list are followed until a diagnosis can be made. To avoid losing babies to follow-up, however, some sort of test can be administered when the newborns are still available for screening, that is, in the nursery.

In order to determine whether a given test is appropriate for screening purposes, one must clearly distinguish between screening and diagnosis. One way to distinguish the two is to think of diagnosis as the process of confirming a specific impairment in an individual. Screening, on the other hand, subdivides a population into two groups of individuals: (1) those who probably are unimpaired, and (2) those who probably are impaired. As a result of screening, the

---

*This material originally appeared in *The Auditory Brainstem Response* by J. T. Jacobson (Ed.) (pp. 317–334). San Diego: College-Hill Press, 1985. It has been adapted for this publication.

second group is referred for diagnosis. Consequently, a good screening test is one that ensures with very high probability that those individuals who pass are not impaired. Remember, these individuals will not be referred for diagnosis! A good diagnostic test, however, is one that ensures with very high probability that those who fail truly have the impairment or disease in question.

The suitability of a given test for either diagnostic or screening purposes will depend on its operating characteristics, which, in turn, are determined by the way the results are interpreted. These characteristics can be quantified, and the test can be rendered more suitable for screening by manipulating the interpretation of the findings.

THE OPERATING CHARACTERISTICS OF A TEST

There are two main operating characteristics of a test. The first is *sensitivity* and denotes the probability that truly impaired individuals will fail the test. The second is *specificity* and designates the probability that truly unimpaired individuals will pass the test. When a test operates at 90 percent sensitivity, 9 out of 10 truly impaired individuals will fail the test. When the same test operates with 90 percent specificity, 9 of 10 truly unimpaired individuals will pass the test.

Figure 2–1 shows a four-box matrix, sometimes called a *decision matrix*, which can clarify these operating characteristics. Each box in the matrix corresponds to a test result, whereas (A) designates the number of impaired individuals who fail the test (i.e., true positives), (B) the number of unimpaired individuals who fail the test (i.e., false positives), (C) the number of impaired individuals who pass (i.e., false negatives), and (D) the number of unimpaired individuals who pass the test (i.e., true negatives). The percent sensitivity of the test is determined by dividing the number of impaired individuals who fail by the total number of impaired individuals—A/A + C—and multiplying by 100. Percent specificity is determined by taking the ratio of the number of unimpaired individuals who pass to the total number of unimpaired individuals—D/B + D—again multiplying by 100.

Consequently, the percent sensitivity is also the true positive rate, and the reciprocal is called the *false-negative rate*. The percent specificity is the true negative rate, and the reciprocal is called the *false-positive rate*. A test with 95 percent sensitivity has a false-negative rate of 5 percent. In other words, there is a 5 percent probability that truly impaired individuals will pass a test having 95 percent sensitivity. If the same test happens to have a specificity of 80 percent, it will have a false-positive rate of 20 percent, meaning that there is a 20 percent chance that truly unimpaired individuals will fail the test.

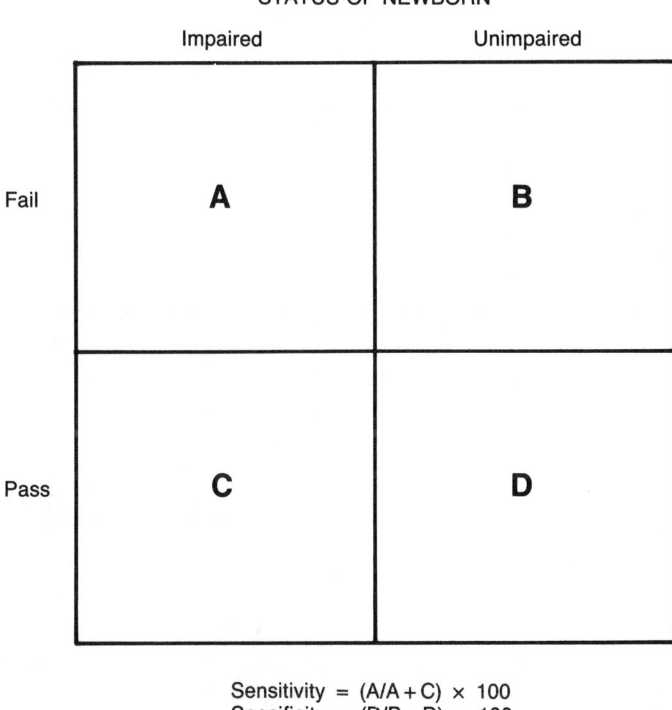

Figure 2–1. A decision matrix demonstrating the computation of a test's operating characteristics. Sensitivity is the ratio of true positives (A) to the total number of impaired newborns (A + C). Specificity is the ratio of true negatives (D) to the total number of unimpaired newborns (B + D). False positives are represented by B, and false negatives are represented by C.

THE CUTOFF SCORE

It is important to understand the implications of choosing the test score that will serve as the ''cutoff'' between pass and fail. On the basis of this choice, a given test will operate with a certain sensitivity and specificity. Moreover, a change in the cutoff score will have a predictable influence on these operating characteristics.

Figure 2–2 shows the distribution of thresholds for unimpaired and impaired newborns who coexist in a hypothetical target population. A cutoff score of 40 dB nHL is represented by the vertical line B. Those who score to the right of this cutoff will fail the test, and those who score at 40 dB nHL or less will pass. Clearly, using this cutoff, all

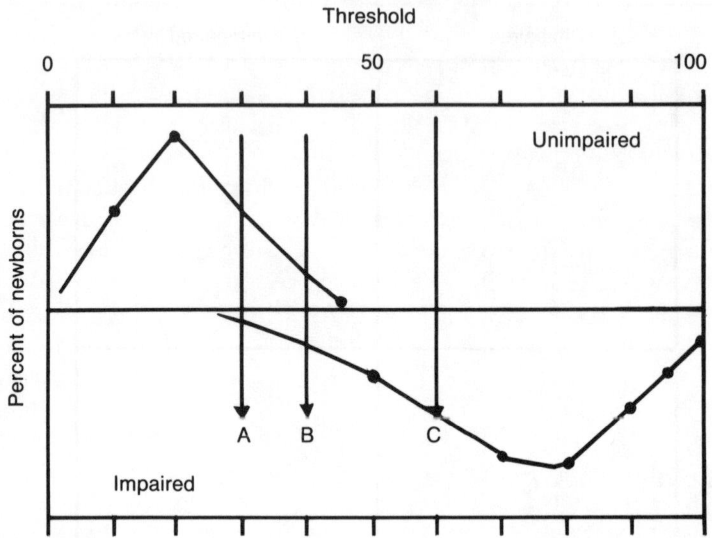

Figure 2–2. Hypothetical distributions of thresholds for unimpaired (top) and impaired (bottom) newborns. Screening cutoff points representing 30 dB nHL (A), 40 dB nHL (B), and 60 dB nHL (C) are as vertical lines. See text for explanation.

the impaired newborns will fail, and the false-negative rate will be very low. With this cutoff, then, the test is operating with high sensitivity. However, a significant proportion of the unimpaired newborns will also fail with this cutoff score, and the false-positive error rate will be correspondingly high because of the reduced specificity.

Adjusting the test cutoff point toward the impaired newborns to line C (60 dB nHL) will markedly increase specificity and decrease sensitivity. This is because none of the unimpaired babies will now fail the test, but a larger proportion of impaired newborns will pass with this cutoff. It is important to note that this change will result unavoidably in a much lower false-positive rate and a higher false-negative rate.

Moving the cutoff point toward the unimpaired newborns will have just the opposite effect. Sensitivity will increase because the probability increases that an impaired baby will fail the test. As a direct result, fewer unimpaired babies will pass and specificity decreases. Accordingly, this adjustment of the cutoff will increase the false-positive rate and decrease the false-negative rate.

Since the main objective in screening is to maximize the confidence in negative results, a cutoff score close to the unimpaired newborns should be selected if we want to eliminate even mild hearing loss. By now it should be apparent that this alteration will have predictable consequences. By increasing the confidence in the negative result, we are decreasing the confidence in the positive result. In other words, the false-positive error rate will inherently be increased.

Therefore, the increase in the false-positive rate associated with an increase in the sensitivity of a test is difficult to avoid. If we wish to rule out only moderate to severe loss, the overlap between the two populations in Figure 2–2 will be reduced. In other words, it may be possible to increase specificity without a marked reduction in test sensitivity. This will reduce the false-positive error rate, but the identification of newborns having mild congenital hearing loss is sacrificed.

THE INFLUENCE OF THE PREVALENCE OF IMPAIRMENT

It is important to remember that these test characteristics are based on probabilities, and, as a result, they may be only indirectly related to clinical outcome. That is, there is a tendency to view these probabilities in clinical terms, and this can lead to pertinent misconceptions. The most pertinent misconception is that sensitivity and specificity will change when the test is administered to different populations. Quite possibly, this notion stems from the practice of equating the false-positive rate with the so-called over-referral rate. When a test is understood to have 90 percent specificity, it follows that it also has a 10 percent false-positive rate. However, this does not mean that 10 percent of those who fail the test will be unimpaired (i.e., over-referrals).

The over-referral rate carries a markedly different connotation in terms of clinical outcome. It is the reciprocal of the *predictive value of a positive test result* and is equal to the ratio of the number of unimpaired individuals who fail the test to the total number of individuals who fail. The most important fact to remember is that the over-referral rate is markedly influenced by the prevalence of the impairment in the population being tested, but the false-positive rate is not, assuming the same cutoff point is used. Therefore, the over-referral rate can change markedly when the false-positive rate of a test does not change at all. The reason is that the sensitivity and specificity of a test do not change when the prevalence of impairment changes. Consequently, the false-positive and false-negative rates do not change.

As an example of these principles, another decision matrix is shown in Figure 2–3. This time a hypothetical population of 1000 newborns is depicted, for which 25 percent are truly impaired. In other words, the prevalence of impairment is 25 percent. If we assume for discussion purposes that a test operates with 95 percent sensitivity and 90 percent specificity, 238 of the 250 truly impaired newborns will fail and 675 of the 750 truly unimpaired newborns will pass. Consequently, the screen will wrongly classify 12 of the impaired newborns and 75 of the unimpaired newborns. Let's take a closer look at these findings. The decision matrix also shows that a total of 315 newborns failed the screen, and 238 (76 percent) were

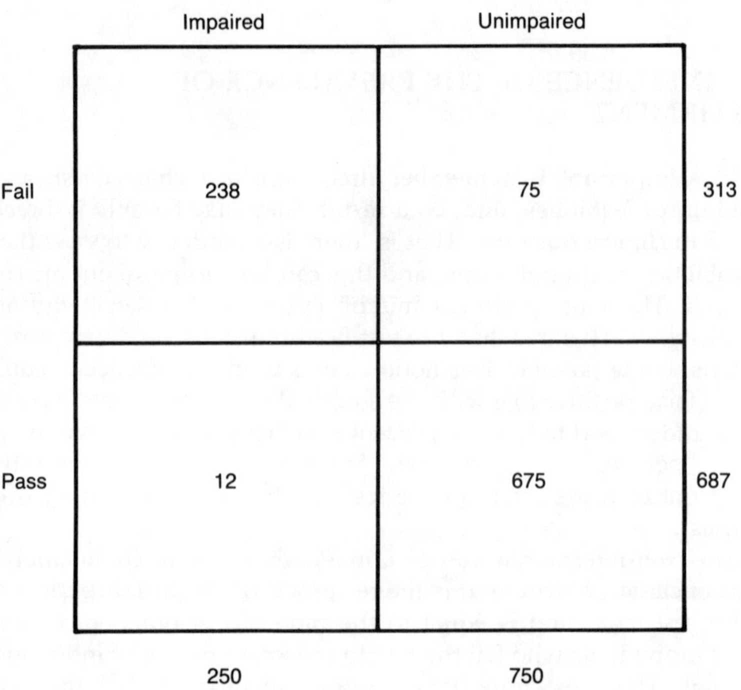

Figure 2–3.   A decision matrix showing the screening results for a hypothetical population of 1,000 newborns of which 25 percent are impaired. The over-referral rate would equal the ratio of false positives (75) to the total number of failures (315). The under referral rate would be the ratio of false negatives (12) to the total number of passes (687). The reciprocals of these two ratios are the predictive value of a positive and negative test result, respectively.

truly impaired; the remaining 75 were unimpaired. That is, the predictive value of a positive screen was 76 percent, and the *over-referral rate* was 24 percent. In the same manner, a total of 687 newborns passed the screen, and, of these, 675 (98 percent) were truly unimpaired; the remaining 12 were impaired. Therefore, the predictive value of a negative result for this population was 98 percent, and the *under-referral* rate was only 2 percent.

What happens if the same screening test is administered to a population of 1000 newborns in which the frequency of occurrence of congenital hearing loss is much lower? Table 2–1 gives the answer for a prevalence of impairment ranging from 1.5 to 5 percent, which includes the range of reported values. The top section of the table illustrates the consequences of using a 30 dB nHL cutoff, which *hypothetically* corresponds to 98 percent sensitivity and 90 percent specificity. The middle and bottom sections, respectively, represent the estimates based on moving the cutoff point toward the impaired newborns to 45 and 60 dB nHL. The assumption is made that the intent is to rule out moderate to severe impairment; therefore, moving the cutoff toward the impaired newborns increases specificity without a marked reduction in sensitivity.

If the top section of the table is entered at 2.5 percent prevalence, we see that approximately 12 percent of newborns will fail the test. Based on the presumed sensitivity and specificity, 25 of the failures are true positives and 98 are false positives. Consequently, the over-referral rate would be 80 percent! Sound familiar? We can now do one of two things. We can either use a higher cutoff or test a population having a different prevalence. If we use the same cutoff and test a population where the prevalence is only 1.5 percent, 11.3 percent will fail, which is composed of 15 true positives and 99 false positives. This translates to an over-referral rate of 87 percent! If the same cutoff is used with a 5 percent prevalence group, the over-referral rate will fall to 66 percent. It is apparent, then, that the number of over-referrals does not necessarily indicate that the test is inaccurate. Very high over-referral rates can be expected when the prevalence of impairment is very low, even though the test is performing very well. Moreover, when the same cutoff point is used to screen populations having a 1.5 percent versus a 5.0 percent prevalence, over-referrals will markedly increase, but the proportion of failures will change very little.

If, instead, we change the cutoff to 45 dB nHL and test the same 2.5 percent population, we can see from the middle section of Table 2–1 that only 7.3 percent will fail and the over-referral rate will fall to 67 percent. The bottom frame of the table shows that moving to a cutoff of 60 dB nHL with a 2.5 percent prevalence will result in 4.4 percent failures and 45 percent over-referrals.

Table 2–1.   A Breakdown of Screening Results for a Hypothetical Population of 1000 High-Risk Newborns

98% Sensitivity, 90% Specificity—30 dB Cutoff

Prevalence	Abn	Nml	tp	fn	fp	tn	OR	PPV	UR	NPV	EFF	% fail
1.5	15	985	15	0	99	887	.87	.13	.00	1.00	.981	.113
2	20	980	20	0	98	882	.83	.17	.00	1.00	.902	.118
2.5	25	975	25	1	98	878	.80	.20	.00	.999	.902	.122
3	30	970	29	1	97	873	.77	.23	.00	.999	.902	.126
3.5	35	965	34	1	97	869	.74	.26	.00	.999	.903	.131
4	40	960	39	1	96	864	.71	.29	.00	.999	.903	.135
4.5	45	955	44	1	96	860	.68	.32	.00	.999	.904	.140
5	50	950	49	1	95	855	.66	.34	.00	.999	.904	.144

97% Sensitivity, 95% Specificity—45 dB Cutoff

Prevalence	Abn	Nml	tp	fn	fp	tn	OR	PPV	UR	NPV	EFF	% fail
1.5	15	985	15	0	49	936	.77	.23	.00	1.00	.950	.064
2	20	980	19	1	49	931	.72	.28	.00	.999	.950	.068
2.5	25	975	24	1	49	926	.67	.33	.00	.999	.951	.073
3	30	970	29	1	49	922	.63	.38	.00	.999	.951	.078
3.5	35	965	34	1	48	917	.59	.41	.00	.999	.951	.082
4	40	960	39	1	48	912	.55	.45	.00	.999	.951	.087
4.5	45	955	44	1	48	907	.52	.48	.00	.999	.951	.091
5	50	950	49	2	48	903	.49	.51	.00	.999	.951	.096

97% Sensitivity, 98% Specificity—45 dB Cutoff

Prevalence	Abn	Nml	tp	fn	fp	tn	OR	PPV	UR	NPV	EFF	% fail
1.5	15	985	14	1	20	965	.58	.42	.00	.999	.980	.034
2	20	980	19	1	20	960	.51	.49	.00	.999	.980	.039
2.5	25	975	24	1	20	956	.45	.55	.00	.999	.980	.044
3	30	970	29	1	19	951	.40	.60	.00	.999	.979	.048
3.5	35	965	34	1	19	946	.36	.64	.00	.999	.979	.053
4	40	960	38	2	19	941	.33	.67	.00	.998	.979	.058
4.5	45	955	43	2	19	936	.31	.69	.00	.998	.979	.062
5	50	950	48	2	19	931	.28	.72	.00	.998	.979	.067

KEY:	Abn	abnormal
	Nml	normal
	tp	true positives
	fn	false positives
	tn	true negatives
	OR	over-referral rate
	PPV	positive predictive value
	UR	under-referral rate
	NPV	negative predictive value
	EFF	overall efficiency
	%fail	overall percentage who fail

SUMMARY AND DISCUSSION

It is important in clinical terms to be mindful of the relationship between the operating characteristics of a test, the selection of the pass-fail cutoff point, and the prevalence of the impairment in the population being screened. These factors have a substantial influence on the predictive value of positive and negative screening results. Moreover, it is this author's contention that these principles can explain the varying screening results of different investigators.

For example, a comment can be made about the operating characteristics of the ABR as a screening test. Invariably, investigators report a very low under-referral rate, meaning that very few if any impaired newborns pass the ABR screen. We now know that this indicates very high test sensitivity. It is not unreasonable to assume, then, that the ABR operates at approximately 98 percent sensitivity when a cutoff score close to the unimpaired newborns is used (i.e., 30 or 40 dB nHL). Specificity is more difficult to estimate, but there are a few clues. Presumably, the incidence of moderate to severe impairment in the NICU graduates is almost 5 percent, and, with this prevalence, most investigators report that between 10 and 20 percent failed the screen and about half of these were over-referrals. This would correspond to a specificity of between 90 and 95 percent!

These estimates directly relate to the concern over the proportion of over-referrals on ABR screening. Clearly, the number of over-referrals can be substantial, even though the test is operating at maximum efficiency. Over-referrals will depend on the cutoff point used and the prevalence of impairment in the population tested. If the cutoff point is very low, such as the 25 dB nHL cutoff used by Shannon, Felix, Krumholz, Goldstein, and Harris (1984), the over-referral rate will soar; especially if newborns outside the NICU are screened, thereby lowering the prevalence of impairment even more.

Clearly, a thorough understanding of the principles of screening and test selection is paramount to planning screening programs for high-risk newborns.

Editor's Note: The cost of the test instrument and the expenditures to carry out the screening program are also of prime consideration in test selection. These issues are addressed in an early section of Chapter 10.

REFERENCES

Northern, J. L., and Downs, M. P. (1974). *Hearing in children*. Baltimore: Williams and Wilkins.

Shannon, D. A., Felix, J. K., Krumholz, A., Goldstein, P. J., and Harris, K. C. (1984). Hearing screening of high-risk newborns with brainstem auditory evoked potentials: A follow-up study. *Pediatrics, 73*, 22–26.

Thorner, R. M., and Remein, Q. R. (1982). Principles and procedures in the evaluation of screening for disease. In J. B. Chaiklin, I. M. Ventry, and R. F. Dixon (Eds.), *Hearing measurement: A book of readings* (2nd ed.). Reading, Massachusetts: Addison-Wesley.

Chapter **3**

The Development and Outcome of the High-Risk Register

Katherine Pike Gerkin

Twenty years have passed since the concept of screening infants for hearing loss was first described (Downs and Sterritt, 1964). Although screening infants for hearing loss proved to be a feasible means of identifying severe hearing deficits in infants, the evolution of programs has been slow until recently. This recent proliferation of hearing screening programs is primarily due to technical advances and increased awareness of the advantages of early identification and the impact on speech and language development.

HISTORY

Ideally every newborn should be screened for hearing loss. Realistically, we are not approaching that goal very quickly, because hearing screening must, in most cases, be implemented on a more conservative scale. At the very least, we must screen those children we know from experience to be ''at risk'' for hearing loss.

The method used in early identification has not been and is not presently without controversy. One widely used approach to infant screening is the use of a high-risk register designed to flag those infants at greater risk for hearing loss than the normal population.

Richards and Roberts (1967) reported that a high-risk register, to be efficient, should identify a disease that is 14 times more prevalent in the register than in the general population. The high-risk register for deafness meets this criteria. The biggest advantage of using a high-risk register lies in the fact that only 10 percent of a total population needs to be screened to identify 65 percent of hearing-impaired babies. This saves both time and money.

In 1969, a National Committee was formed of representatives from the Academy of Pediatrics, the Academy of Ophthalmology and Otolaryngology, and the American Speech and Hearing Association and was charged with making recommendations for Newborn Infant Hearing Screening. After reviewing several studies, Feinmesser and Tell (1976), Cunningham (1971), McCulloch (1973), Mencher (1974) (see Chapter 1 for descriptions of studies), the Joint Committee identified five factors (see Table 3–1) to be determined by means of history and physical examination that should be the basis for referral for an audiological evaluation by 2 months of age.

In 1981, the Joint Committee revised and expanded the high-risk criteria to include seven conditions that pose a threat to a newborn's hearing. The following is a list of the high-risk factors described by the 1982 Joint Committee:

1. A family history of childhood hearing impairment.
2. Congenital perinatal infection (e.g., cytomegalovirus, rubella, herpes, toxoplasmosis, syphilis).
3. Anatomic malformations involving the head or neck (e.g., craniofacial syndromal abnormalities, overt or submucous cleft palate, morphological abnormalities of the pinna).
4. Birthweight less than 1500 gm.
5. Hyperbilirubinemia at levels exceeding indications for exchange transfusion.
6. Bacterial meningitis, especially from *Haemophilus influenzae*.
7. Severe asphyxia, which may include infants with Apgar scores of 0–3 or who fail to institute spontaneous respiration by 10 minutes and those with hypotonia persisting to 2 hours of age.

Table 3–2 lists the same factors in a mnemonic fashion termed the *ABCD's of Deafness* (Gerkin, 1984).

These risk factors provide a base for an effective hearing screening program. An understanding of each factor will aid the audiologist in implementing a screening program ensuring proper follow-up procedures for diagnosing hearing loss in infants.

RISK FACTORS

Asphyxia

Asphyxia might commonly be called *suffocation*. It is a condition in which there is a lack of oxygen and an increased carbon dioxide

Table 3–1. The 1972 Joint Committee High-Risk Register

---

1. History of hereditary childhood hearing impairment.

2. Rubella or other non-bacterial intrauterine fetal infection (e.g., cytomega-lovirus infections, herpes infection).

3. Defects of ear, nose, or throat. Malformed low-set or absent pinnae; cleft lip or palate (including submucous cleft); any residual abnormality of the otorhinolaryngeal system.

4. Birthweight less than 1500 gm.

5. Bilirubin level greater than 20 mg/100 ml serum.

Table 3–2. ABCD's of the 1982 High-Risk Register for Deafness

---

A. Asphyxia

B. Bacterial meningitis

C. Congenital or perinatal infections

D. Defects of the head or neck

E. Elevated bilirubin

F. Family history

G. Gram birthweight < 1500

---

tension in the blood and tissues. Anoxia is a term used to describe the end result of lack of oxygen. Anoxia may occur in the fetus or after birth for a variety of reasons. Regardless of the cause, prenatal or perinatal anoxia can result in either central or peripheral respiratory failure.

Asphyxia is directly related to the gestational age and birthweight of an infant. Preterm infants are more likely to experience anoxic episodes than are full-term infants (MacDonald, 1967).

Apgar Score. The Apgar score is probably the best immediate indication of an infant's condition at birth (Apgar and James, 1962). The Apgar score examines heart rate, respiration effort, muscle tone, reflex response, and color at 1 minute and 5 minutes following birth. Each category is given a score of 0, 1, or 2. A total score of 10 would indicate the infant is in the best possible condition. Table 3–3 provides details of the Apgar scoring system. The low Apgar score at 1 minute is an indication of asphyxia, whereas the low 5-minute score is an index of the likelihood of death or neurological residual (Vaughn, McKay, and Behrman, 1979).

Table 3–3. Apgar Scoring

Sign	0	1	2
Heart rate	Absent	Below 100	Over 100
Respiratory effort	Absent	Slow, irregular	Good, crying
Muscle tone	Limp	Some flexion of extremities	Active motion
Response to catheter in nostril	No response	Grimace	Cough or sneeze
Color	Blue, pale	Body pink, extremities blue	Completely pink

From R. E. Behrman and V. C. Vaughn, III (1983). *Nelson textbook of pediatrics* (12th ed.) (p. 336). Philadelphia: W. B. Saunders Company. Reprinted by permission.

Hearing Loss. A ready supply of oxygen is essential to the organ of Corti. Hearing loss as a result of asphyxia has been described by Simmons (1980) and D'Souza, McCartney, Nolan, and Taylor (1980). Simmons suggests that anoxia may be the underlying cause for most neonatal deafness. This is a difficult premise to substantiate because of the many associated problems a severely asphyxiated infant usually experiences.

The hearing loss manifested by asphyxia is sensorineural in nature with a steep slope in the high frequency range (Simmons, 1980). There is also an extremely high incidence of middle ear disease in neonates who require long term intubation as a result of asphyxia or respiratory distress (Berman, Balkany, and Simmons, 1978). Thus, neonates with a history of asphyxia need both careful high frequency hearing screening and continued otological follow-up for otitis media.

Bacterial Meningitis

Meningitis results from bacteria in the blood. Although *H. influenzae* is the most common agent in older children and adults, the most common organisms causing the disease in newborns are *Escherichia coli* and Group B streptococci (Krugman and Katz, 1981; Vaughn et al., 1979). Early onset of infection in neonates usually results from bacteria in the amniotic fluid or maternal genital tract. Late onset (after the first week of life) can be contracted from a variety of environmental sources.

Bacterial meningitis in the newborn is difficult to recognize. The diagnosis is complicated by symptoms that are nonspecific and resemble many kinds of sepsis seen in newborns. Symptoms include fever, lethargy, respiratory distress, jaundice, anorexia, vomiting, and diarrhea.

Bacterial meningitis develops in approximately 1 of 2500 live births (Feigan and Dodge, 1976). The mortality rate for neonatal meningitis is 40 to 75 percent, despite early intervention and antibiotics. A high proportion of survivors have serious neurologic sequelae (Koops and Battaglia, 1980; Krugman and Katz, 1981).

Hearing Loss. Hearing loss results from passage of the infection from the meninges to the inner ear via the cochlear aqueduct and along vessels and nerves from the internal auditory meatus (Paparella and Suguira, 1967). Sensorineural deafness occurs in 7 to 35 percent of infected patients (Berlow, Caldarelli, Matz, Meyer, and Harsch, 1980; Finitzo-Hieber, 1982; Vernon, 1967). Mild cases of hearing loss as well as unilateral losses have been documented, but bilateral, severe sensorineural hearing loss is typical of bacterial meningitis. Rosenthall and Kankkunen (1980) report approximately one fourth of all patients with meningitic hearing loss enjoy partial or complete recovery in one or both ears. In contrast, Berlow and associates (1980) suspect hearing loss due to meningitis to be progressive in nature. Persistent follow-up is essential due to the variable nature concerning hearing loss.

Congenital or Perinatal Infections

Congenital or perinatal infections are major causes of morbidity and mortality in the newborn. It is estimated that 2 percent of fetuses are infected in utero and 10 percent are infected during the first month of life (Vaughn et al., 1979). The fetus may acquire disease from the maternal bloodstream across the placenta from infected amniotic fluid or by direct contact with infected maternal tissue in the birth canal. Infections are termed *congenital* if acquired in utero, *perinatal* if acquired at the time of birth, and *postnatal* if contracted after birth during the neonatal period. Infection of the fetus or neonate can result in reabsorption of the embryo, abortion, still-birth, malformation, intrauterine growth retardation, premature birth, acute disease, or asymptomatic infection with neurological sequelae (Klein, Remington, and Marcy, 1983; Vaughn et al., 1979).

There is a specific group of infectious diseases associated directly with hearing loss in infants. These infections are referred to as the TORCH complex, T for toxoplasmosis, R for rubella, C for cytomegalovirus, H for herpes, and O for others (hepatitis B virus, enterovirus, mumps, listeria, gonorrhea, streptococcus, syphilis). It is estimated that 1 to 5 percent of all deliveries are infected by one of the TORCH agents, resulting in a minimum of 400 deaths per year and at least 2000 persons who are left with significant sequelae (Nahmias, 1974). Subtle or similar clinical signs make these infectious diseases difficult to distinguish. Furthermore, many of the diseases are asymptomatic at birth but can later result in serious defects.

Toxoplasmosis

Toxoplasmosis is caused by the protozoan parasite *Toxoplasma gondii*. Although first described in animals in 1908 by Nicolle and Maneaux, toxoplasmosis did not make an impact on medicine as a disease entity in humans until 1937.

It is estimated that 3300 of the 33 million infants born each year in the United States have congenital infection. Most of these children are asymptomatic at birth but have sequelae of the infection developing later in life (Remington and Desmont, 1983).

Toxoplasmosis is transmitted to the fetus from the maternal bloodstream. It is not known how a pregnant woman acquires the organism. However, there is some evidence that uncooked meat or contact with cat feces containing oocysts may be possible sources. It is likely that this only occurs when the infection is acquired during pregnancy. The fact that only primary infection results in affected infants is critical to the prevention of the disease. If acquired infection during pregnancy was prevented, the disease could be almost entirely eradicated. Congenital toxoplasmosis is manifested by chorioretinitis, cerebral calcification, psychomotor retardation, hydrocephalus or microcephaly, and convulsions.

Hearing Loss. Campbell and Clifton (1950) described moderate progressive hearing loss in three of four family members affected with acquired toxoplasmosis. In another 4-year follow-up study of newborns with toxoplasmosis, 17 percent had hearing loss (Abrams, 1977).

Syphilis

Although not specifically recognized under the TORCH acronym, syphilis is considered here so as not to be overlooked as a congenital infection that causes hearing loss.

There has been a dramatic decline in the number of cases of congenital syphilis since the advent of penicillin therapy. However, there is truth in the saying that as a control program approaches eradication of that disease, it is likely that the control program rather than the disease will be eradicated. Approximately 64,875 cases of syphilis are reported annually (U.S. Department of Health, Education and Welfare, Sexually Transmitted Diseases: Statistical Letter, 1978); although it is estimated that only one of every three cases is actually reported (Fleming, Brown, Donohue, and Branigan, 1970). Syphilis is caused by the spirochete *Treponema pallidum*. Humans are the only host. The fetus is usually infected in utero by transplacental passage of the organism, but infection may occur from contact with an infectious lesion during passage through the birth canal. For decades, it was thought that only after the 18th week was the placental barrier vulnerable to syphilis (Strome, 1977). More recent evidence obtained by pathological examination of aborted fetuses prior to 12 weeks gestation showed the organism to be present. However, no inflammatory response was present unless gestation was 15 weeks or more in duration (Krugman and Katz, 1981). Penicillin treatment of the mother during pregnancy generally ''cures'' the infant in utero, although some inflammation may already have occurred. Untreated primary syphilis in pregnant women results in infected fetuses 70 to 100 percent of the time (Krugman and Katz, 1981). Undiagnosed cases of maternal syphilis result in a 50 percent mortality rate in utero and in neonates (Strome, 1977).

The manifestations of congenital syphilis are multiple and severe. The signs and symptoms appear both as early (the first 2 years of life) and late manifestations, occurring anytime thereafter. A congenitally infected infant may appear perfectly normal at birth. Early manifestations include bony changes, rhinitis, rash, anemia, and jaundice. Hutchinson's teeth, mulberry molars, and sensorineural hearing loss are late problems.

Hearing Loss. Hearing loss is not usually apparent at birth but occurs around puberty. Patterns of deafness show variations dependent upon time of onset and rapidity of progression (Kerr, Smyth, and Cinnamond, 1973), but typically the hearing loss is sudden, bilateral, symmetrical, profound, and with no accompanying vestibular symptoms (Karmody and Schuknecht, 1966). Unfortunately, in the case of congenital syphilis, one can expect poor hearing function and limited use of hearing aids due to neural atrophy (Black et al., 1971).

Rubella

Rubella is an acute infectious disease caused by rubella virus. A large epidemic in the 1960s left 10,000 to 20,000 children handicapped. Although this country has not seen rubella in epidemic proportions since the 1960s, the disease persists.

The number of rubella immunizations has decreased as public anxiety has lessened and the length of immunity of the vaccine has been questioned. It appears that in some cases, vaccine only provides immunity for 8 to 12 years (Vernon and Klein, 1982).

Humans are apparently the only host for rubella virus; thus, the disease is maintained in nature through cycling among humans. Rubella virus is generally transmitted person to person by respiratory droplets. Maternal viremia leads to infection of the placenta and fetus. The virus can affect virtually all fetal organs. The classic rubella syndrome is characterized by intrauterine growth retardation, cataracts, microcephaly, deafness, congenital heart disease, and mental retardation.

If the fetus is infected during the first month of pregnancy, the chances of developing congenital rubella defects are 50 percent. The incidence then drops to 22 percent affected the second month, and 6 to 10 percent affected in the third, fourth, and fifth months of pregnancy (Pumper and Yamashiroya, 1975).

Hearing Loss. Hearing loss can occur from infection any time during pregnancy, but it is more common when the fetus is infected during the first trimester.

Koningsmark and Gorlin (1976) and others have described a "cookie bite" audiogram in relation to rubella deafness, with the greatest degree of loss in the mid-frequency range from 500 to 2000 Hz. Severe to profound sensorineural hearing loss usually results, although middle ear anomalies have also been described (Sando and Wood, 1971).

Cytomegalovirus

Cytomegalovirus (CMV) infects approximately 1 percent of newborns, and as many as 60 to 80 percent of the United States population acquire CMV by midadult life. The virus may be congenitally or perinatally acquired. The most common congenital route is thought to be transplacental, whereas perinatal infection is commonly acquired as the baby passes through an infected birth canal.

The effects of CMV vary from severe central nervous system destruction to asymptomatic excretion of the virus. The classic congenitally infected symptomatic infant is characterized by an enlarged liver and spleen, hyperbilirubinemia, thrombocytopenia with petechiae on purpura, cerebral calcifications, microcephaly, chorioretinitis, deafness, and psychomotor retardation (Weller and Hanshaw, 1962). The prognosis for severely affected infants is grim. As many as 25 percent of symptomatic infants die within the first 3 months of life (Pass, Stagno, Myers, and Alford, 1980; Weller and Hanshaw, 1962). Of the remainder, 60 to 75 percent will have intellectual or developmental impairment, one third will have hearing impairment, one third neuromuscular disorders, and some will exhibit visual impairment (Berenberg and Nankervis, 1970).

The overall clinical picture of the asymptomatic infant is less severe, and long-term outcome of mild affects due to the virus are still under investigation.

Hearing Loss. The incidence of hearing loss in symptomatic infants is thought to be approximately 30 percent (Pass et al., 1980). The probability of hearing loss in asymptomatic infants varies (Harris, Ahlfors, Ivarsson, Lernmark, and Svanberg, 1984; Reynolds et al., 1974; Stagno et al., 1977), but is probably the most common irreversible sequela of asymptomatic CMV.

Hearing loss attributable to CMV is sensorineural in nature, but the pattern and severity are extremely variable. The hearing loss ranges from mild to profound and may be unilateral or bilateral. Progressive hearing loss is also well documented (Dahle, McCollister, Stagno, Reynolds, and Hoffman, 1979; Gerkin and Northern, 1984; Pass et al., 1980).

Herpes Simplex Virus

Herpes simplex virus (HSV) causes one of the most common sexually transmitted diseases. It is the second most common viral infection in pregnant women and is surpassed only by CMV. The most common mode of transmission to the infant is during the birth process if the mother is actively infected. Even when the mother is asymptomatic, the virus may be present in the genital tract and may infect the fetus. There is some evidence that HSV may occasionally be transmitted transplacentally or postnatally (Nahmias, Keyserling, and Kerrick, 1983).

The prognosis for infants with HSV is grim. The infection often becomes disseminated or involves the central nervous system, and there is a high mortality rate. Survivors are likely to have severe sequelae.

Hearing Loss. Although reports of HSV and hearing loss are scant, histopathological studies show that HSV infects the sensory cells of the labyrinth (Veltry, Wilson, Sprinkle, Rodman, and Kavesch, 1981). Any infant with HSV infection should have careful audiological follow-up.

Defects of the Head and Neck

Anomalies associated with craniofacial and skeletal syndromes are numerous. The defects range from very subtle abnormalities to overt manifestations. Neonates with head and neck defects include craniofacial syndromal abnormalities, overt or submucous cleft palate, or any morphologic abnormalities of the pinna.

The variety of abnormalities as well as the associated hearing loss are too numerous to discuss in detail. For detailed descriptions of the various head and neck disorders, the reader is referred to the books by Jaffe (1977), Northern and Downs (1984), or most textbooks that include treatment of otolaryngology or birth defects. Attention should be drawn to the fact that many of the more subtle disorders (e.g., low set ears, ear tags) are often noted at birth but are not referred for otological or audiological follow-up.

Hearing Loss. Any anomaly of the pinna may also have an associated middle ear anomaly (Jaffe, 1977), and any infant exhibiting such a defect deserves audiological evaluation.

Hyperbilirubinemia

Hyperbilirubinemia is a condition in which there is an excessive amount of bilirubin in the blood, and it can be neurotoxic to the infant at certain concentrations. Jaundice (yellowing), the resulting clinical manifestation, is observed during the first week of life in approximately 60 percent of term infants and 80 percent of pre-term infants. Normally, bilirubin levels peak at 3 days of life in a term baby and approximately 5 days of life in a premature infant. The bilirubin levels then decline steadily. Toxicity is thought to occur in cases in which the serum bilirubin levels continue to climb.

As red blood cells break down at the end of their normal useful life, hemoglobin is released in the plasma and converted to bilirubin. The bilirubin is then bound to plasma albumin and transported to the liver where an enzyme ''conjugates'' or joins it together with a substance in the body to form a detoxified product. The now ''conjugated'' bilirubin is generally excreted normally through the intestinal tract.

Any factor that interferes with transporting the bilirubin to the liver or reduces or prohibits the liver from metabolizing the bilirubin can lead to increased serum levels. Hemolytic disease, hemorrhages, and polycythemia are a few of the more common causes of hyperbilirubinemia. Other pathological conditions (i.e., anoxia, infection, drugs) may also contribute to toxic serum levels and enhance the ability of bilirubin to cross the blood–brain barrier and enter brain tissue. Kernicterus is a neurological syndrome resulting from the deposition of bilirubin in brain cells. Cell destruction specifically in the area of the basal ganglia and hippocampus were found in cases of kernicterus. More recently, staining of bilirubin has been found to be more widely distributed throughout the brain in animal studies (Levine, Fredericks, and Rapoport, 1982).

Many factors contribute to a physician's decision as to whether or not an infant requires exchange transfusion. Unfortunately, there is no clear-cut answer as to what is potentially toxic, and autopsies of premature infants show bilirubin staining at fairly low concentrations (Maisels, 1982).

The Committee of Fetus and Newborn (1977) of the Academy of Pediatrics suggested the levels shown in Table 3–4 for exchange transfusion. This should be used as a guide by the audiologist in determining whether or not to place a child on the high-risk register.

Hearing Loss. Hearing loss associated with hyperbilirubinemia was much more prevalent before exchange transfusions became common practice to treat the disease. Hyman and colleagues (1969) reported multiple abnormalities in 405 infants with hemolytic disease and hyperbilirubinemia. Hearing impairment was found in 4.2 percent, or 17 infants. In 10 of the 17, or 59 percent, hearing impairment was the only abnormality, with a higher incidence in those infants who were premature. The losses ranged in severity from mild to profound and included both bilateral and unilateral sensorineural losses.

Simmons (1980) cited hyperbilirubinemia as the most common sequela of anoxia causing deafness. It is important to note that many babies who are hyperbilirubinemic have other complicating pathological factors that could cause or contribute to a hearing loss. Severe sensorineural hearing loss was attributed to hyperbilirubinemia in one child seen at the author's clinic who had mistakenly been given hemolized blood during a transfusion.

Family History

Hereditary deafness includes a large number of syndromes as well as deafness with no associated anomalies. More than 50 types of hereditary hearing loss have been delineated.

Congenital deafness may be inherited in a variety of ways. The basic patterns of inheritance, greatly simplified here, are dominant inheritance, recessive inheritance, and X-linked inheritance.

Dominant Inheritance

In dominant inheritance, a single abnormal gene is sufficient to produce deafness. One parent has an affected gene, which can be passed to the offspring. In the case of dominant inheritance, there is a 50 percent chance that each child will manifest the hearing loss. Hereditary deafness inherited in this manner occurs in approximately 10 percent of the cases (Fraser, 1976).

Table 3–4. Suggested Exchange Transfusion Levels According to Birthweight

Birthweight (gm)	Serum Bilirubin Level for Exchange Transfusion (mg/100 ml)	
	Normal Infants	*Abnormal Infants*
<1,000	10.0	10.0
1,001–1,250	13.0	10.0
1,251–1,500	15.0	13.0
1,501–2,000	17.0	15.0
2,001–2,500	18.0	17.0
>2,500	20.0	18.0

From Committee of Fetus and Newborn (1977). *Standards and recommendations for hospital care for newborn infants* (6th ed.) (p. 95). Evanston, IL: American Academy of Pediatrics. Copyright 1977 by the American Academy of Pediatrics. Reprinted by permission.

Hearing Loss. Often the hearing loss is not present at birth and develops later.

Recessive Inheritance

In recessive inheritance, both parents appear essentially normal but by chance, carry a defective gene. Each offspring has a 25 percent chance of receiving the defective gene from both parents and manifesting the defect. There is also a 25 percent chance for each child not to inherit the gene from either parent, in which case he or she will be totally normal. Finally, there is a 50–50 chance of receiving only a single defective gene and thus becoming a carrier.

Hearing Loss. Recessive hearing impairment is the most common form of inherited deafness. Approximately 40 percent of profound childhood deafness is attributed to autosomal recessive inheritance. The degree and pattern of hearing loss is variable, but it is generally most severe in the high frequencies, resulting in what is often termed a ''corner audiogram.''

X-Linked

Normal females have two X-chromosomes, whereas males have one X and one Y chromosome. In X-linked inheritance, the mother carries the faulty gene on one X chromosome. There is a 50 percent chance that she will pass the affected gene to each son who will manifest the defect. There is a 50 percent chance that each daughter will inherit the gene but will be a carrier and not manifest the abnormality. Approximately 1 to 3 percent of hereditary deafness is due to this type of transmission.

Hearing Loss. The hearing loss is probably not present at birth but develops in early infancy and progresses with varying rapidity (Livan, 1961; Mohr and Mageroy, 1969).

Birthweight Less than 1,500 Grams

Low birthweight has long been considered a risk factor in hearing loss. It is certainly well documented that premature infants have a high incidence of hearing loss, but there is little agreement on the relative incidence of hearing loss in this group or on the actual cause of the hearing impairment.

The problem of diagnosis of the hearing loss lies in the fact that premature infants undergo more associated health problems in their early stages than do full-term infants. Among the more commonly seen problems associated with a premature infant are anoxia, hyperbilirubinemia, an increase in bacterial and viral infections, and treatment with ototoxic drugs. Any of these factors alone may cause deafness. In combination with low birthweight, the effects may be more frequent.

There is no doubt that there is a relationship between prematurity and deafness. What that relationship actually is remains to be resolved through additional research.

Hearing Loss. The hearing loss in low birthweight infants is generally sensorineural, high frequency, and steeply sloping (Davey, 1962). There is also a high correlation between low birthweight infants and otitis media, especially in cases of prolonged intubation (Berman, Balkany, and Simmons, 1978).

Clark and Conry's (1978) study of 204 low birthweight babies revealed 5 percent with sensorineural hearing loss. All these 11 babies also had elevated bilirubin levels. McDonald (1967) reported 19 cases of hearing loss in 1066 infants with birthweights under 4 lb (1800 gm). There was a significant correlation between postnatal hypoxia and the hearing loss.

Drillen (1964) tested 433 premature children of school age and found 17.5 percent to have some hearing deficit. In 42 percent, there was no obvious cause of the hearing defect.

SUMMARY

An understanding of the high-risk factors provides the audiologist with a basic tool to assist in diagnosing hearing loss in infants. The high-risk register cannot identify every conceivable cause of deafness. At present, it provides a basic format to assist in implementing an infant screening program and ultimately identifying hearing loss in newborns.

We should look forward to the day that all infants can be screened and thus have an equal chance for early diagnosis and habilitation.

REFERENCES

Abrams, I. F. (1977). Nongenetic hearing loss. In B. F. Jaffe (Ed.), *Hearing loss in children*. Baltimore: University Park Press.

Apgar, V., and James, L. (1962). Further observations on the newborn scoring system. *American Journal of Diseases of Children, 104*, 419.

Behrman, R. E., and Vaughn, V. C. (1983). *Nelson textbook of pediatrics* (12th ed.). Philadelphia: W. B. Saunders Company.

Berenberg, W., and Nankervis, G. (1970). Long-term follow-up of cytomegalic inclusion disease of infancy. *Pediatrics, 46*, 403–410.

Berlow, S. J., Caldarelli, D. D., Matz, G. J., Meyer, D. H., and Harsch, G. G. (1980). Bacterial meningitis in sensorineural loss. *Laryngoscope, 90* (9), 1445–1452.

Berman, S. A., Balkany, T. J., and Simmons, M. A. (1978). Otitis media in the neonatal intensive care unit. *Pediatrics, 62*, 198–202.

Black, F. O., Bergstrom, L., Downs, M. P., et al. (1971). *Congenital deafness: A new approach to early detection through a high risk register*. Boulder, CO: Colorado Associated University Press.

Campbell, A. M. G., and Clifton, F. (1950). Adult toxoplasmosis in one family. *Brain, 73*, 281–290.

Clark, B. R., and Conry, R. F. (1978). Hearing impairment in children with low birthweight. *Journal of Auditory Research, 18*, 4.

Committee of Fetus and Newborn. (1977). *Standards and recommendations for hospital care for newborn infants* (6th ed.). Evanston, IL: American Academy of Pediatrics.

Cunningham, G. C. (1971). Conference on newborn hearing screening. *Proceedings, summary, and recommendations of a conference on newborn hearing and early identification of hearing impairment conducted at Oakland, California.* Berkeley, CA: California State Department of Public Health, Bureau of Maternal and Child Health.

Dahle, A. J., McCollister, F. P., Stagno, S., Reynolds, D. W., and Hoffman, H. E. (1979). Progressive hearing impairment in children with congenital CMV. *Journal of Speech and Hearing Disorders, 44*, 220.

Davey, P. R. (1962). Hearing loss in children of low birthweight. *Journal of Laryngology and Otolaryngology, 76*, 274–277.

Downs, M. P., and Sterritt, G. M. (1964). Identification audiometry for neonates: A preliminary report. *Journal of Auditory Research, 4*, 69–80.

Drillen, C. M. (1964). *The growth and development of the prematurely born infant.* Edinburgh: E. and S. Livingstone, Ltd.

D'Souza, S. W., McCartney, E., Nolan, M., and Taylor, I. G. (1981). Hearing, speech, and language in survivors of severe perinatal asphyxia. *Archives of Disease in Childhood, 56*, 245–252.

Feigin, R. D., and Dodge, P. R. (1976). Bacterial meningitis: Newer concepts of pathophysiology and neurologic sequelae. *Pediatric Clinics of North America, 23*, 3.

Feinmesser, M., and Tell, L. (1976). Evaluation of methods for detecting hearing impairment in infancy and early childhood. In G. T. Mencher (Ed.), *Early identification of hearing loss.* Basel: S. Karger.

Finitzo-Hieber, T. (1982). Auditory brainstem response: Its place in infant and audiological evaluations. *Seminars in Speech, Language, and Hearing, 3,* (1), 76–87.

Fleming, W. L., Brown, W. N., Donohue, J. F., and Branigan, P. W. (1970). National survey of venereal disease treated by physicians in 1968. *JAMA, 211,* 11.

Fraser, G. R. (1976). *The causes of profound deafness in childhood.* Baltimore: The Johns Hopkins University Press.

Gerkin, K. P. (1984). The high-risk register for deafness. *ASHA, 26* (3), 17–23.

Gerkin, K. P., and Northern, J. L. (1985). Special case studies: Cytomegalovirus. In J. T. Jacobson (Ed.), *The auditory brainstem response* (pp. 395–396). San Diego: College-Hill Press.

Harris, S., Ahlfors, K., Ivarsson, S., Lernmark, B., and Svanberg, L. (1984). Congenital cytomegalovirus infection and sensorineural hearing loss. *Ear and Hearing, 5*(6), 352–355.

Hyman, C. B., Keaster, V., Hanson, V., Harris, I., Sedgwick, R., Wursten, H., and Wright, A. R. (1969). CNS abnormalities after neonatal hemolyte disease or hyperbilirubinemia. *American Journal of Diseases of Children, 117,* 395–405.

Jaffe, B. F. (1977). Middle ear and pinna anomalies. In B. F. Jaffe (Ed.), *Hearing loss in children* (p. 294). Baltimore: University Park Press.

Karmody, C. S., and Schuknecht, H. F. (1966). Deafness in congenital syphilis. *Archives of Otolaryngology, 83,* 18–26.

Kerr, A., Smyth, G. D., and Cinnamond, M. J. (1973). Congenital syphilitic deafness. *Journal of Laryngology and Otolaryngology, 87,* 1–12.

Klein, J. O., Remington, J. S., and Marcy, S. M. (1983). Current concepts of infections of the fetus and newborn infant. In J. S. Remington and J. O. Klein (Eds.), *Infectious diseases of fetus and newborn infant* (pp. 1–26). Philadelphia: W. B. Saunders Company.

Konigsmark, B. W., and Gorlin, R. J. (1976). *Genetic and metabolic deafness.* Philadelphia: W. B. Saunders Company.

Koops, B. L., and Battaglia, F. C. (1980). The newborn infant. In C. H. Kempe, H. K. Silver, and D. O'Brien (Eds.), *Current pediatric diagnosis and treatment* (p. 78). Los Altos, CA: Lange Medical Publications.

Krugman, S., and Katz, S. (1981). *Infectious diseases of children.* St. Louis: The C. V. Mosby Company.

Levine, R. L., Fredericks, W. R., and Rapoport, S. I. (1982). Entry of bilirubin into the brain due to opening of the blood–brain barrier. *Pediatrics, 69,* 3.

Livan, M. (1961). Contributo alla conoscenza della sordita creditarie. *Archivio Italiano Otolaryngologia, 72,* 331–339.

Maisels, M. J. (1982). Jaundice in the newborn. *Pediatrics in Review, 3,* 10.

McCulloch, B. J. (1973, September). Paper read at the Tenth International Conference on Birth Defects, Vienna, Austria.

McDonald, A. (1967). Children of very low birthweight. *MEIV Research Monograph No. 1,* Heinemann, London.

Mencher, G. T. (1974). Infant hearing screening: The state of the art. *Maico Audiological Library Series,* Vol 12, No 7.

Mohr, J., and Mageroy, K. (1960). Sex-linked deafness of a possibly new type. *Acta Genetics, 10,* 54–62.

Nahmias, A. J., Keyserling, H. L., and Kerrick, G. M. (1983). Herpes simplex. In J. S. Remington and J. O. Klein (Eds.), *Infectious diseases of the fetus and newborn infant* (p. 639). Philadelphia: W. B. Saunders Company.

Nahmias, A. J. (1974). The TORCH complex. *Hospital Practice, 9,* 65–72.

Northern, J. L., and Downs, M. P. (1984). *Hearing in children* (3rd ed.). Baltimore: Williams and Wilkins.

Paparella, M. M., and Suguira, S. (1967). The pathology of suppurative labyrinthitis. *Annals of Otology, Rhinology, and Laryngology, 75,* 554–586.

Pass, R. F., Stagno, S., Myers, G. J., and Alford, C. A. (1980). Outcome of symptomatic congenital cytomegalovirus infection results of long-term longitudinal follow-up. *Pediatrics, 66* (5), 758–762.

Pumper, R. W., and Yamashiroya, H. M. (1975). *Essentials of medical virology.* Philadelphia: W. B. Saunders Company.

Remington, J. S., and Desmont, G. (1983). Toxoplasmosis. In J. S. Remington and J. O. Klein (Eds.), *Infectious disease of the fetus and newborn infant* (pp. 144–148). Philadelphia: W. B. Saunders Company.

Reynolds, D. W., Stagno, S., Stubbs, K. G., Dahle, A. J., Livingston, M. M., Saxon, S. S., and Alford, C. A. (1974). Inapparent congenital cytomegalovirus infection with elevated cord IgM levels. *New England Journal of Medicine, 290,* 7.

Richards, I. D. G., and Roberts, C. J. (1967). The at-risk infant. *Lancet, 2,* 711–714.

Rosenthall, V., and Kankkunen, A. (1980). Hearing alterations following meningitis; 1. Hearing improvement. *Ear and Hearing, 1,* 185.

Sando, I., and Wood R. P. (1971). Congenital middle ear anomalies. *Otolaryngology Clinics of North America* (Symposium), 4, 311, 435.

Simmons, F. B. (1980). Patterns of deafness in newborns. *Laryngoscope, 90,* 448–453.

Stagno, S., Reynolds, D. W., Amos, C. S., Dahle, A. J., McCollister, F. P., Mohindra, O. D., Ermocilla, R., and Alford, C. A. (1977). Auditory and visual defects resulting from symptomatic and sub-clinical congenital CMV and toxoplasma infections. *Pediatrics, 59,* 669–678.

Strome, M. (1977). Sudden and fluctuating hearing losses. In B. F. Jaffe (Ed.), *Hearing loss in children* (pp. 478–479). Baltimore: University Park Press.

Vaughn, V. C., III, McKay, J. R., and Behrman, R. E. (1979). *Nelson textbook of pediatrics,* (11th ed., pp. 393–395). Philadelphia: W. B. Saunders Company.

Veltry, R. W., Wilson, W. R., Sprinkle, P. M., Rodman, S. M., and Kavesch, D. A. (1981). Implication of virus in idiopathic sudden hearing loss: Primary infection of reactivation of latent viruses. *Otolaryngology and Head and Neck Surgery, 89* (1), 137–141.

Vernon, M. (1967). Meningitis and deafness: The problem, its physical, audiological, and educational manifestations in children. *Laryngoscope, 77,* 1856–1874.

Vernon, J., and Klein, N. (1982). Hearing impairment in the 1980's. *Hearing Aid Journal, 35*(5), 17–21.

Weller, T. H., and Hanshaw, J. B. (1962). Virological and clinical observation of cytomegalic inclusion disease. *New England Journal of Medicine, 266,* 1233–1344.

Chapter **4**

The Crib-o-gram in Neonatal Hearing Screening*

George R. Marcellino

BACKGROUND

The reported estimates of the incidence of severe to profound hearing loss in neonatal populations varies widely. Northern and Downs (1974) reported that 1 in 2000 children have severe congenital hearing impairment at birth. Feinmesser (1976) found an incidence of 1 in 709 for a population of 17,731 newborns, whereas Downs and Hemenway (1969) reported an incidence of 1 in 1000. Simmons, McFarland, and Jones (1979) found that 1 in 819 in the well-baby nursery and 1 in 57 in the neonatal intensive care unit had severe hearing impairment, for an over-all incidence figure of 1 in 329. Recently, using the brainstem evoked response, Galambos and Galambos (1979) reported an incidence of severe hearing loss in 1 of 50 infants who required intensive care during the neonatal period. Looking at infants at risk for hearing loss determined by a high-risk registry, Downs (1978) estimates the incidence of hearing impairment to be 1 in 50 for those considered at risk.

There is little doubt that untreated moderately severe to profound hearing losses preclude normal cognitive, social, speech and language development (Luterman and Chasin, 1970; Northern and Downs, 1974; Shaw, Chandler, and Dale, 1978). Early detection

---

*This material originally appeared in three publications of *Hearing Instruments*, 30(6), 12–15 (1979); 32(6), 12–15 (1981); and 32(8), 10–12 (1981). San Diego: Harcourt, Brace, Jovanovich, Inc. It has been adapted for this publication.

markedly improves the prognosis for speech and language development through provision of appropriate medical, surgical, or habilitative therapy (Luterman and Chasin, 1970; Northern and Downs, 1974; Ruben, 1978; Shaw, Chandler, and Dale, 1978). Therefore, early detection of congenital hearing impairment is a worthwhile goal.

Techniques for the auditory screening of neonates may be divided into the following three categories: (1) physiological, (2) high-risk register, and (3) behavioral (motor) responses.

1. *Physiological techniques:* Electrophysiological techniques, most notably auditory brainstem response and electrocochleography, require highly trained personnel and expensive equipment. Therefore, these techniques may not be cost effective insofar as mass screening is concerned.

Acoustic impedance measurements provide a means of assessing middle ear function by tympanometry, whereas the acoustic reflex may sometimes be used as a predictor of sensorineural hearing loss (Burney, Mauldin, and Crump, 1974). According to Keith (1973), "of 160 stimulus presentations to normal hearing subjects only 30% resulted in a clear stapedial reflex." It was believed that impedance audiometry was not the answer to the problems of mass infant hearing screening.

Measurement of cardiac and respiratory changes associated with acoustic stimulation have been suggested as methods for neonatal screening. According to Gerber (1977), "data on the cardiovascular responses to sound in the infant unfortunately are equivocal at best." With regard to respiration audiometry, Gerber further states that "apparently normal newborns do alter their respiratory patterns following acoustic stimuli, but no correlation has been shown between the level of stimulation and the respiratory pattern or its changes."

2. *High-risk register:* Identification of neonates with hearing impairment through utilization of the high-risk register as suggested by the Joint Committee on Neonatal Hearing Screening has been disappointing. Using the five categories suggested, Feinmesser (1976) reported a false-negative rate of 33 percent.

3. *Behavioral response:* Behavioral response is typically determined by human observation of an infant's behavior following a stimulus from a hand-held source placed in close proximity to the infant. The tester delivers the stimulus and then observes whether or not a change in activity state occurred that was correlated to the stimulus presentation. This technique suffers the disadvantage of undefined criteria for simultaneously monitoring a multitude of possible responses, questionable interobserver reliability, and high false-positive rates. Because the scorer presents the test stimulus and consequently knows when to anticipate a response, a scoring bias is inherently present.

PROTOTYPE CRIB-O-GRAM

To eliminate some of the difficulties encountered with the use of human observers, F. Blair Simmons developed an automated technique, called a Crib-o-gram, to record changes in activity state of neonates. Since the current microprocessor hearing screening instrument is based upon the prototype Crib-o-gram, it is important to understand the design of the original instrument and review the reports of Simmons (1977), Simmons and Russ (1974), and Simmons and associates (1979).

The Equipment

The key element of the Crib-o-gram unit was an extremely sensitive motion-sensing transducer that was placed beneath the infant's crib mattress. The original transducer and the one used in the current model consists of a piezoelectric bimorph mounted on an aluminum disc. The transducer produces a charge proportional to the change in force impressed upon it. The transducer output voltage is amplified and fed to a strip chart recorder, which registers changes in motor activity ranging from small respiratory changes to startle response.

The Crib-o-gram contained a loudspeaker placed at the foot of the crib. Automatically a 1-second narrowband noise stimulus with a center frequency at 3000 Hz was presented at 92 dB. Neonatal motor activity was monitored for 12 seconds before (baseline), 1 second during, and 2.5 seconds following the stimulus. This test cycle was repeated at regularly controlled intervals over a 24-hour period. Typically, 30 stimuli were presented. In addition, a silent control was administered at each tenth trial and served as a cross-check on the scorer's accuracy and for assessment of random neonatal motor activity.

Scoring

On the strip chart, a timing marker located above the activity waveform produced by the activity on the infant (Fig. 4–1) indicated that the stimulus was presented at that time. The scorer measured waveforms before and after the stimulus marker in order to determine whether or not a response to the auditory stimulus had occurred.

The criteria used to determine a response follow:

1. If the amplitude of the largest positive peak minus the most negative peak in a 3.5-second post-stimulus onset interval is at least two times or one half the amplitude of the largest peak-to-peak

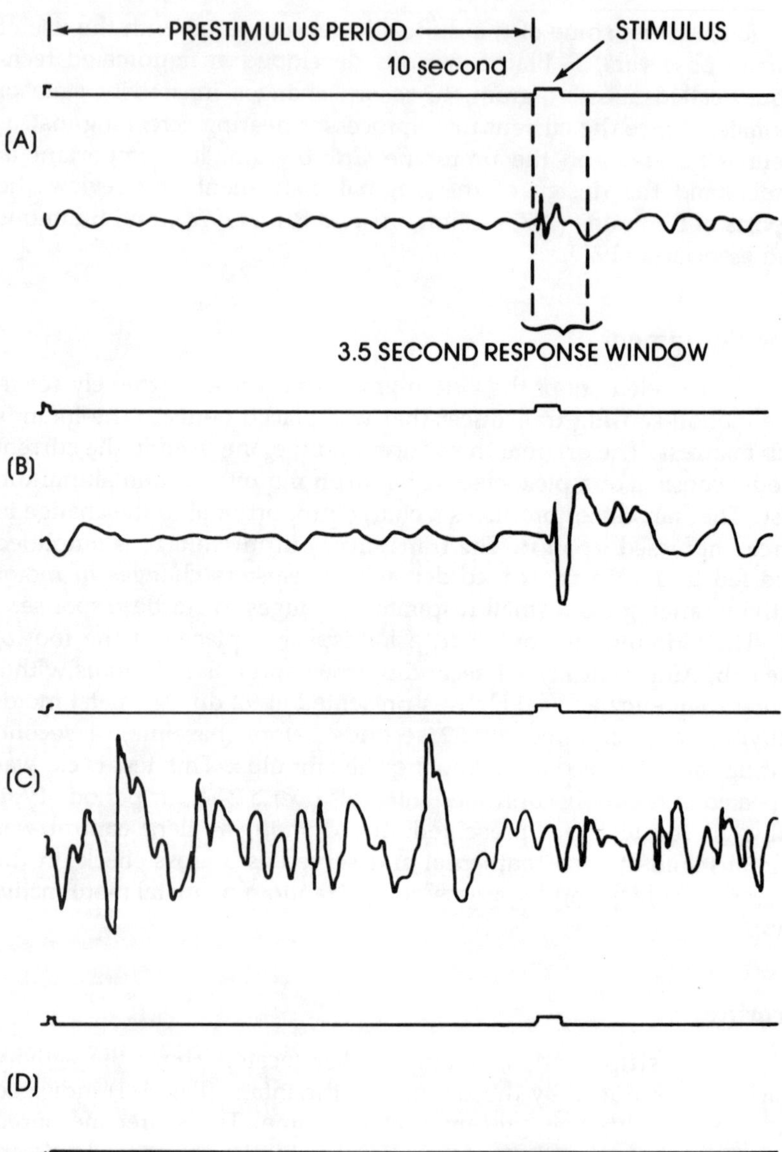

Figure 4–1. Time windows for Crib-o-gram trial data collection and analyses. The waveforms represent: *A*, Periodic respiratory pattern and response; *B*, slight activity and response; *C*, unacceptably high level of activity; and *D*, unacceptably low level of activity or baby absent from crib.

amplitude in the pre-stimulus interval, a response was considered to have occurred.

2. If the number of changes in direction per second (frequency of movement) in the post-stimulus period were at least two times or less than one half the number of changes in direction per second in a pre-stimulus period, a response was counted.

3. A 10 percent positive response rate was considered a screening pass.

Random Versus Real Responses

By comparing neonatal responsitivity to auditory stimuli and silent control periods, Simons and colleagues (1979) reported that it was possible to establish the rate of random neonatal responses. Figure 4–2 illustrates the number of neonatal responses to real and silent tests as a function of duration after stimulus onset. The results indicate a random average response rate of 4.6 percent and an average real response rate of 36 percent for infants in the neonatal intensive care unit. The data were obtained from normally hearing babies and were based on 2787 real and 308 silent tests. Baseline activity that tended to produce low real-to-random ratios was eliminated from scoring.

Figure 4–2 shows that the stimulus response latency interval is an important variable. Noteworthy is the fact that, as the time window for post-stimulus activity analysis increases, there is an increasing probability of incorrectly scoring random changes in activity as positive responses. Therefore, the two and one half-second limit for monitoring a response was selected.

Accuracy

Screening accuracy is generally assessed in terms of false-positive and false-negative error. A false-positive error occurs when a baby fails the screening and is shown at follow-up to have normal hearing. A false-negative error occurs when a hearing impaired infant incorrectly passes initial screening.

The false-positive error rate for the well-baby population in a longitudinal study conducted at Stanford University was 8 percent, whereas the error for the intensive care population was 20 percent. For the two populations of infants who passed the screening and for whom the follow-up was available, only one hearing-impaired baby was reported to have been missed by the screening.

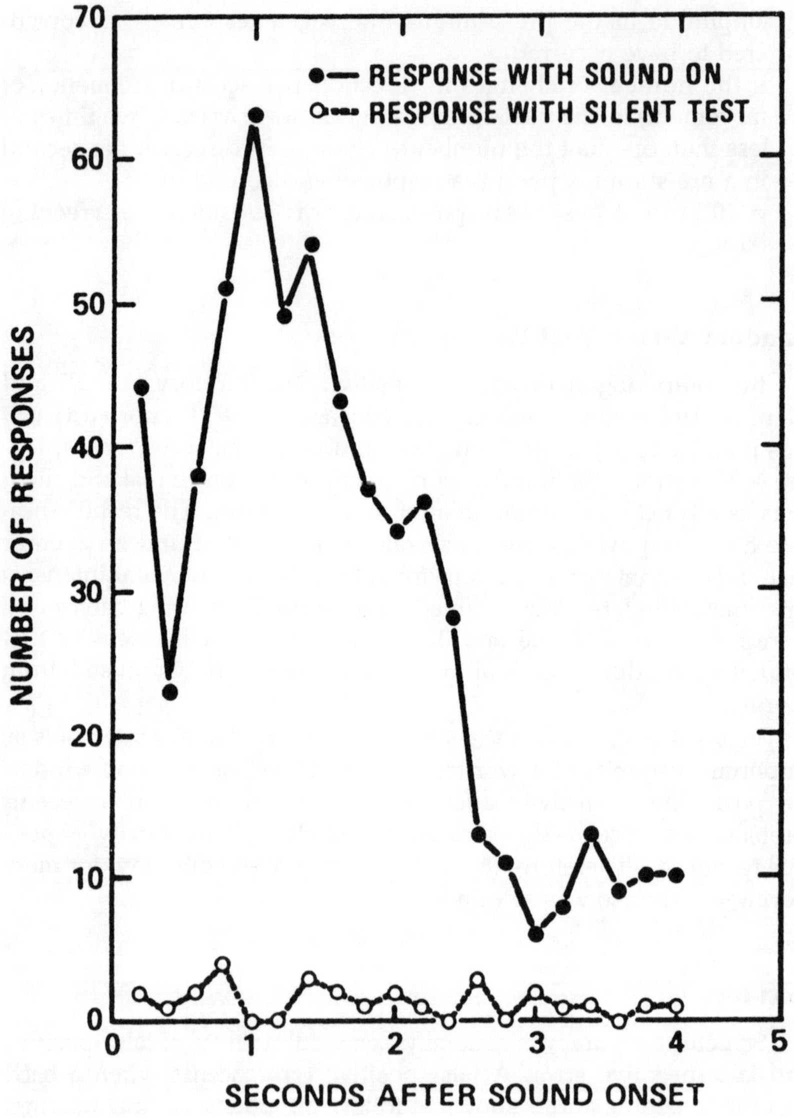

Figure 4–2.   Neonatal responsivity as a function of time after stimulus onset with responses to real and silent tests as parameters. From F. B. Simmons, W. H. McFarland, and F. R. Jones (1979). An automated hearing screening technique for newborns. *Acta Otolaryngologica*. Copyright 1979 by Almqvist and Wiksell. Reprinted by permission.

The false-positive error rate of 20 percent for the intensive care unit population was judged to be too large for implementation of a cost-effective screening program. Therefore, the major design objective of a future microprocessor-based system was to minimize the false-positive error rate while not sacrificing an extremely low false-negative error rate.

Several sources of error were identified with respect to manually scoring strip chart recordings of neonatal motor activity. These include the following:

Scoring strip chart waveforms was a difficult visual pattern recognition task.

There was an a priori clinical bias to fail infants.

There was an inefficient use of the data provided in the strip chart waveform. With criteria of two times the post-stimulus peak amplitude with reference to the pre-stimulus range for a response, both 1.9 times and 1.0 times are both treated as nonresponses.

There was an unfounded assumption that the probability of obtaining 1 of 10, 2 of 20, or 3 of 30 responses for a 10 percent criterion for pass are equivalent.

RESEARCH AND DEVELOPMENT OF THE MICROPROCESSOR

Scoring Algorithm

A standard method of maximally using the information available in each trial is provided by the theory of signal detectability. Although this model is typically applied in the areas of visual and auditory detection, it is exquisitely applicable to the problem at hand. The source of the data for algorithm development were strip charts of neonatal motor activity obtained from the Stanford University Medical Center Crib-o-gram study. The waveforms were converted to digital signals by means of an optical character recognition device and analog-to-digital converter. The data were then in appropriate form for manipulation and analysis by a PDP 11/34 computer.

Statistical Approach

The following assumptions were used in the development of the scoring algorithms:

1. The screening system measures neonatal movement. Measurements can be made on the movement transducer signal that can be used to infer a state of activity in the neonate.

2. When a normal hearing neonate is exposed to a loud auditory stimulus, the activity state of the neonate may change. Although the most likely change is from a less active state to one of greater activity, the opposite change might also occur.

3. Exposure to the auditory stimulus will not always result in a perceptible change in activity. Changes in activity will also result from other stimuli, either external (i.e., visual, tactile) or internal (i.e., dreams, hunger). However, for normal hearing neonates, a change in activity state is more likely to occur immediately following an auditory stimulus than in an absence of such a stimulus.

Because babies vary in mass and motion and transducers and amplifiers can vary in gain, the decision algorithms do not search for absolute amounts of activity but rather look for changes in activity following an auditory stimulus relative to activity preceding the stimulus. The method analyzed a 10-second period before presentation of an auditory stimulus and a 3.5-second period following onset of the stimulus. Four basic measurements descriptive of activity state were made in each of the two periods (Table 4–1).

The set of eight numbers is then used to calculate four statistical descriptions of change in activity from the pre-stimulus period to the post-stimulus period. These four statistics are summarized in Table 4–2.

In describing the amplitudes of the peaks, we chose to add to the manually scored Crib-o-gram method, measures of maximum amplitude, range, mean peak-to-peak amplitude and the variance of these amplitudes. These measures were chosen because they are standard measures for distributions and their sampling distribution is expected to be more stable than the distribution of the maximum amplitude.

The statistics H and D were used because they had already been used in the manually scored program. The statistics T^* and F^* were chosen because they are the natural ways of asking whether or not the mean or variance of distribution has changed.

The next step in the procedure was to convert each of the four members, T^*, F^*, H, and D into one number representing the probability that the neonate had heard an auditory stimulus. This is done by four different likelihood functions derived from empirical data. If there is no change in mean behavior from pre- to post-stimulus, T is expected to be distributed as Student's t distribution with $N_a + N_b - 2$ degrees of freedom. If post-stimulus behavior is significantly different from pre-stimulus behavior, large values of T will be much more likely than would be predicted by the t distribution.

Thus, having calculated a value of T for a trial, we can now calculate the probability of getting such a value of T if there were not a true change in behavior and thus calculate the probability that behavior has actually changed.

Similarly, F^* is intended to determine whether or not the variance of peak-to-peak amplitudes is the same in the post-stimulus

Table 4–1. Statistical Calculations Used During the Pre-Stimulus (Baseline) and Post-Stimulus Periods (MCOG refers to the Manually Scored Crib-O-Gram Method.)

In the pre-stimulus (baseline) period, calculate:

1. The mean value of the absolute magnitude of the peak-to-peak amplitudes M_b
2. The variance of the absolute magnitudes of the peak-to-peak amplitudes V_b
3. The average number of peaks per second A_b
4. The largest positive peak minus the largest negative peak (i.e., the range of the signal R)

In the post-stimulus period, calculate:

1. The mean value as in the pre-stimulus interval M_a
2. The variance as in the pre-stimulus interval V_a
3. The average number of peaks in the pre-stimulus interval A_a
4. The largest absolute magnitude of peak-to-peak amplitudes L (i.e., that maximum value that is also used in the MCOG method)

---

period as the pre-stimulus period. The statistic F is a measure of the ratio of the two variances. If there is no change in behavior from pre- to post-stimulus, this statistic should be distributed as the analysis of variance F tests with $N_a - 1$ degrees of freedom. Thus, we can, for each value of F, calculate the odds, F*, favoring the hypothesis that variance behavior has changed. The actual calculation of F* from F* and T* from T is done using a series of approximation.

These four probabilities are then multiplied by each other to obtain the total probability that the neonate heard the stimulus. This procedure is then repeated for all the trials. The probabilities represented by each trial are multiplied by one another to provide a number representing the evidence that the child can hear. The logarithm of this number is determined and a value greater than 50 (ß) is considered to be a pass, whereas a number less than 50 is considered to be a screening failure. Determination of the appropriate cutoff value and scaling the final number was partially achieved through trial and error. Figure 4–3 graphically shows the position of the scoring criterion (ß) with respect to baseline random neonatal motor activity and changes in activity in response to an acoustic stimulus.

Through the application of the scoring algorithms to the Stanford strip chart data for children who have received follow-up confirmation of hearing status and application of the scoring method to other independent data bases, it was possible to achieve a false-negative error rate of approximately 5 percent and a false-positive error rate of approximately 12 percent for the neonatal intensive care nursery population.

Table 4–2.   Further Statistical Computations Performed at the End of Each Screening Trial

---

These statistics are:

1. $T = \dfrac{(M_a - M_b)}{\sqrt{V_c \bullet \left(\dfrac{1}{N_a} + \dfrac{1}{N_b} \right)}}$ where $V_c = \dfrac{N_b \bullet V_b + N_a\, V_a}{N_a + N_b - 2}$

and N_b and N_a are the number of peaks in the pre- and post-stimulus intervals, respectively

2. $F = \dfrac{N_a \bullet (N_b - 1) \bullet V_a}{N_b \bullet (N_a - 1) \bullet V_b}$

3. $H = L/R$
4. $D = A_a/A_b$

The statistics T and F are further operated on to obtain the numbers:

T^* = the probability of obtaining a value as large as T under the hypothesis that mean amplitude did not change from pre- to post-stimulus.

F^* = the probability of obtaining a value as large as F under the hypothesis that the variance of peak-to-peak amplitudes did not change from pre- to post-stimulus

---

CURRENT MICROPROCESSOR CONTROLLED CRIB-O-GRAM

The use of a PDP/11 computer was impractical insofar as neonatal hearing screening is concerned. Thus, the next phase in development was to program a microprocessor system that could score neonatal

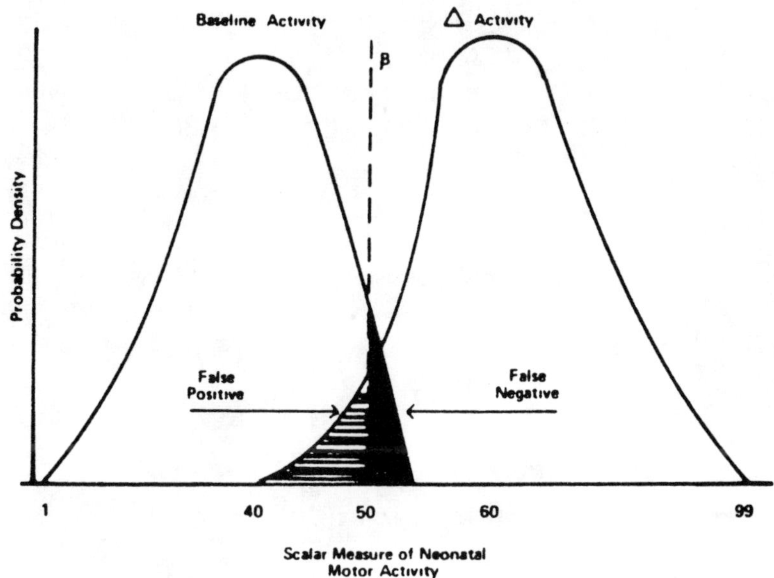

Figure 4–3. Approximate distributions of neonatal motor activity for pre-stimulus (baseline) periods. The abscissa is a log transformation of likelihood ratios obtained for each statistic and then multiplied across 30 trials. Beta (ß) is set at 50 and defines the false-positive and false-negative error rates.

responses the same way as the PDP/11 computer. A description of the microprocessor version of the Crib-o-gram follows.

The device (Fig. 4–4) contains a speaker, which can be placed at the head or foot of the crib, and a motion transducer, which is placed under the mattress. A sound level meter is used to calibrate 92 dB of narrowband noise at the level of the baby's ear.

After initialization of the screening program, the Crib-o-gram unit automatically determines the appropriate behavioral-arousal state for testing. The microprocessor system analyzes 10 seconds of peak-to-peak activity and accepts motion that roughly corresponds to behavioral states of light sleep or quiet wakefulness. If judged appropriate, these 10 seconds of data are stored in random access memory and serve as the trial baseline. If the baseline is deemed inappropriate, the system will resample activity 80 seconds later. After an appropriate baseline is stored, the acoustic stimulus is then automatically generated and neonatal motion is monitored for 3.5 seconds from stimulus onset.

Activity is analyzed by comparing various measures described in detail earlier that characterize the baseline and post-stimulus periods.

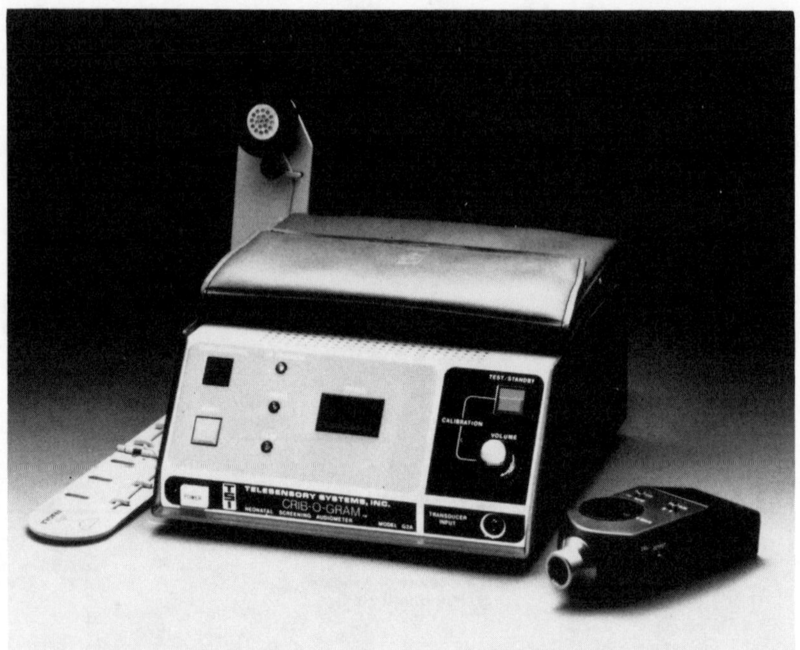

Figure 4–4. Microprocessor controlled Crib-o-gram.

These measures include statistical comparisons of (1) mean values of the absolute magnitudes of the peak-to-peak amplitudes, (2) variance between the two time windows, (3) the average number of peaks in the waveform, and (4) the range of peak-to-peak amplitudes. These statistical results are combined to form a single likelihood ratio (odds estimate), which predicts the probability that changes in neonatal motion are indicative of a response to auditory stimuli. Since a single observation is insufficient to draw accurate conclusions, 30 trials are conducted with their respective likelihood ratios multiplied across all 30 trials to provide the end result.

The Crib-o-gram provides two indicators of screening results. The first is the pass-refer decision, which is displayed automatically on the front of the instrument at the end of the screen. It is determined by the magnitude of the scalar score. The scalar score, a number that ranges from 20 to 99, is the second indicator of results and is an over-all indicator of responsiveness during the 30 trials. It is a probability estimate that the infant has normal hearing. Scalar scores less than 50 are screen failures, whereas scalar scores of 50 or greater are screen passes. Although the probability of hearing impairment is inversely related to the magnitude of the scalar score, no direct relationship between the magnitude of the scalar score and degree of hearing impairment has been established.

An interpretation of scores can be seen from the following example: Suppose two screenings are administered, and a scalar score of 50 is obtained on the first screen and a score of 70 is obtained on the second screen. Both estimates suggest that the newborn is not hearing impaired on a statistical basis. There are numerous possibilities to account for the difference in scores. Determination of the appropriate arousal state varies and threshold values are only approximations. Therefore, the degree of neonatal arousal can be a factor affecting the final score. If days pass between screens, the neonate is really another subject altogether. Maturation, illness, and so on combine to define an entirely different response set. The Crib-o-gram design criteria is robust with respect to these issues, and results are intended to differentiate hearing newborns from hearing-impaired newborns.

Validation Study

To obtain validation information for the Crib-o-gram scoring system, data were collected and analyzed from 1195 Level III intensive care newborns in hospitals throughout the United States and Canada. For 854 of these newborns (Group I), the following data were collected: (1) pass-refer decision, (2) scalar score, (3) screen duration, and (4) diagnostic information when possible.

Data for 341 additional neonates (Group II) were obtained from hospital sites that agreed to follow specific screening and diagnostic protocol. In addition to data collected for Group I, screen-rescreen results were also obtained. All babies who failed the first screen and a random 20 percent of newborns who passed the first screen received auditory brainstem response (ABR) testing in the form of latency-intensity functions for the wave V potential.

Babies who passed ABR received a second Crib-o-gram screen to assess test-retest reliability in terms of false-positive error. The random 20 percent follow-up of Crib-o-gram passes followed by ABR also provided an estimate of false-negative error. Babies who failed ABR testing underwent as many as three additional Crib-o-gram screens to estimate test-retest reliability and false-negative error. Babies who failed ABR testing also received audiological evaluations using conditioned responses or localization responses at 7 months of age or earlier.

Results. Results can be interpreted by observing Group I, Group II, and combined group data. The principal difference between groups is a more rigid follow-up protocol, test-retest results, and random sample diagnostic testing on 20 percent of the "pass" screens for the Group II population.

Of 854 infants screened on a one-time screen basis for referral in Group I, 165 (19.32 percent) failed the screen. Follow-up ABR or behavioral audiometry testing or both confirmed 18 infants (10.97 percent of those referred, 2.1 percent of all tested) with hearing impairment in excess of 30 dB HL. Diagnostic follow-up information was obtained for 34 percent of the "failed" population.

False-negative error occurs when a newborn is judged to be a screen "pass" but is shown to have hearing loss. Although there was no special attention given to sample babies in Group I who passed, there were no reports given of false-negative error.

The results for the 341 neonates in Group II are as follows: (1) screen referrals, 60 (17.65 percent), (2) confirmed hearing impaired, 10 (2.9 percent), (3) false-positive error, 50 (14.7 percent) and (4) follow-up rate of 43 percent. An extremely important finding was that for the 20 percent random sample of newborns who passed the screen, none were found to have thresholds as measured with the ABR procedure of greater than 30 dB in the better ear.

Since the results for those parameters listed are similar for Groups I and II, the data were combined in order to provide better estimates of the Crib-o-gram performance characteristics. Table 4–3 summarizes the data from Group I, Group II, and the combined groups.

Inspection of Table 4–4 for combined date reveals that a total of 28 hearing-impaired newborns were identified from 1195 babies screened (2.34 percent) after follow-up on 36.4 percent of the "failed" population (225 cases). If it is assumed that the cases lost to follow-up were not anatomically or physiologically different from the cases that were successfully followed, the true incidence would be $2.34/0.364 = 6.43$ percent. Being more conservative, the incidence rate was adjusted to 5 percent ± 2 percent. This, in turn, implies that the true false positive after complete follow-up will be in the range of 13.83 to 15.83 percent. Therefore, approximately one of six babies screened will be referred, and approximately one of three referrals will be hearing impaired.

The combined data may be visualized best by plotting the frequency of occurrence of the scalar scores. Figure 4–5 shows this relation. The x's denote individual data for confirmed hearing-impaired subjects. Scalar scores were obtained for 21 of the 28 newborns with hearing losses. Recall that scalar scores less than 50 are screen failures, and scores of 50 or more are screen passes.

Table 4–3.   Data Summary for Group I, Group II, and Combined Populations

	Group I	%	Group II	%	Combined	%
N	854		341		1,195	
Pass	689	80.7	281	82.4	970	81.11
Fail	165	19.32	60	17.6	225	18.83
Confirmed Hearing-Impaired	18	2.1	10	2.9	28	2.34
False Positive	147	17.2	50	14.7	197	16.5
False Negative	0		0		0	
Follow-up	56	34.0	26	43.0	82	36.4
Ratio—Fail/Hearing-Impaired	1:10.9		1:6		1:8	
Adjusted Incidence						5 ± 2%
Adjusted False-Positive Rate						13.83
Adjusted Fail/Hearing-Impaired Rate					1:4	
Sensitivity						86.0
Specificity						94.5

Table 4–4.   Frequency of Hearing Loss in the Better Ear in Categories From Mild to Profound for Newborns Whose Hearing Loss was Detected by Crib-o-gram

Degree of Loss*	Number of Children	%
Mild (27–40 dB HL)	5	18.0
Moderate (41–55 dB HL)	3	11.0
Moderately Severe (56–70 dB HL)	1	4.0
Severe (71–90 dB HL)	2	7.0
Profound (91 dB HL—NR)	17	61.0

*Hearing loss computed as average pure tone thresholds where possible. In other instances, ABR thresholds to click or filtered noise stimuli or average behavioral response level to complex stimuli were used.

The distributions obtained were directly comparable to those derived during the development phase of the microprocessor Crib-o-gram. The average scalar score for those newborns who passed was 79.2, whereas the scalar scores for those who failed and those with confirmed hearing losses averaged 41 and 36.51, respectively. The probability of false-negative error with a scalar score of 79.2 is less than 0.00005.

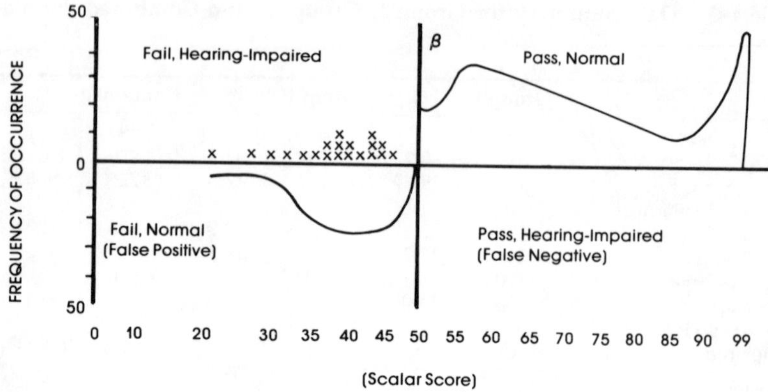

Figure 4–5. Scalar score distributions for 1195 newborns. Each "X" represents a confirmed hearing-impaired child. No false-negative cases were reported.

Table 4–4 summarizes the degree of hearing loss in the better ear. Note that 8 of the 28 confirmed cases have average hearing losses of less than 56 dB HL in the better ear. In the moderate category, one case showed a high-frequency sloping audiogram. The remainder of these newborns (20, or 72 percent) had average thresholds in the better ear in excess of 56 dB HL.

The 2 × 2 matrices in Table 4–5 show the predicted and adjusted outcomes for 1195 tertiary care newborns. There were significant differences between the predicted and adjusted outcomes. Specifically, the Crib-o-gram identified more neonates as hearing impaired than predicted, and the false-positive error rate of 14.83 was not significantly greater than the predicted 12 percent ±2 percent. The only real difference between the expected and adjusted outcomes is the true incidence of hearing impairment. The adjusted incidence of 5 percent ±2 percent falls between the 2 percent incidence reported by Simmons and colleagues (1979) and the 10 percent incidence reported by Galambos and Galambos (1979) for intensive care neonates. False-negative error was assessed by (1) incidental reports, (2) 20 percent random sample of Group II screen passes, and (3) test-retest of confirmed hearing-impaired newborns. No false-negative cases were reported.

Reduction in Interstimulus Interval

The microprocessor design reduced test time from 24 hours for the original instrument to approximately 2.5 to 3 hours. Nevertheless, the time to administer a Crib-o-gram screen is predominantly

Table 4–5.   Expected and Adjusted Outcomes for Crib-o-gram Screening of 1195 Tertiary Intensive Care Newborns

	A. Expected True State			B. Adjusted True State	
	Hearing-Impaired	*Normal*		*Hearing-Impaired*	*Normal*
Crib-o-Gram Decision	20 Fail p (refer, hearing-impaired) = 0.017	143 False-positive p (normal, refer) = 0.120	*Crib-o-Gram Decision*	59.75 Fail p (refer, hearing-impaired) = 0.0500	167.3 p (refer, normal) = 0.140
	1[1] Pass p (pass/ hearing-impaired) = 0.055	1030 Pass p (pass, normal) = 0.862		3.48 Pass p (pass/ hearing-impaired) = 0.054	964.75 Pass p (pass, normal) = 0.809

[1]False-negative error is defined by convention as the number of incorrect decisions divided by the subpopulation of impaired cases.

determined by the time period between stimuli. This time period is called the *interstimulus interval* (ISI).

Concern about habituation arose when reduction of the ISI was considered. With an absence of a specific ISI built into the system, a minimum of 21½ to 25½ seconds still exists between stimuli. This time period consists of a 10-second baseline, a 3½-second response window, and a 8- to 12-second computation period.

Miller and Simmons (1984) reported the results of a study developed by Marcellino in 1981 to assess the effects of reducing the ISI on the scalar score and pass-refer ratio of the Crib-o-gram screens. At Stanford University Medical Center and Oakland Children's Hospital, 494 infants were divided into two groups, depending on whether or not a specific ISI was used between stimuli presentation. It was hypothesized that the average scalar score for babies who pass and those who fail would not vary as a function of prolonged or diminished intertrial intervals. The results can be seen in Table 4–6. There was no difference in pass-fail ratio or the average scalar score between groups. Thus, the average Crib-o-gram screening duration was reduced from approximately 2.5 hours to less than 1 hour.

DISCUSSION

To screen newborns for hearing loss, Simmons used the familiar stimulus-response behavioral model to objectively assess neonatal responses to auditory stimuli by recording mattress motion on a

Table 4–6.   Results of Crib-o-gram With and Without Interstimulus Interval

	Diminished Intertrial Interval		Prolonged Intertrial Interval	
Sample size	149		345	
Pass	129	(86.5%)	295	(85.5%)
Refer	20	(13.5%)	52	(14.5%)
Average scalar score	62.5		64.9	
Standard deviation	18.11		18.36	

From K. Miller and F. Blair Simmons (1984). A retrospective and an update on the Crib-o-gram neonatal hearing screening audiometer. *Seminars in Hearing,* 5(1), 55. Copyright 1985 by Thieme–Stratton, Inc. Reprinted by permission.

strip-chart recorder. These motion recordings could later be scored to determine whether or not a change in activity had occurred in response to an auditory stimulus. During the multicenter, National Institutes of Health sponsored longitudinal study designed to assess the efficacy of the Crib-o-gram screening method, it was readily apparent that manually scoring strip charts was time consuming and no simple task. In addition, interscorer reliability was only fair.

A new solution was offered. A microprocessor-controlled Crib-o-gram (Model G2A) was designed that was able to determine the ''appropriate'' arousal state based on pre-established high- and low-threshold values, control administration of the stimuli with infinite patience, and complete these tasks in a reasonable period of time.

The Crib-o-gram was not intended as a substitute for diagnostic assessment, nor was it intended to identify hearing-impaired newborns more accurately than diagnostic tests. The Crib-o-gram was designed pragmatically as a cost-effective approach to identifying newborns with significant hearing loss before leaving the hospital.

Numerous reports, including those of Galambos and Galambos (1979); Stein, Ozdamar, Kraus, and Paton (1983); and Durieux-Smith, Picton, Edwards, Goodman, and MacMurray (1985) have dealt with the issue of determining hearing sensitivity in the newborn and identification of the newborn at risk for hearing impairment using auditory brainstem response technology. Durieux-Smith and associates (1985) compared Crib-o-gram screening results with results of ABR testing. Such comparisons should be interpreted with caution. Crib-o-gram was intended as a screening instrument to identify those newborns who were likely to be hearing impaired and would require additional diagnostic testing. Crib-o-gram was designed to be inexpensive and easy to operate. ABR, on the other hand, can be used as a sophisticated diagnostic test. To date, it is expensive to administer and requires trained personnel to interpret the test results.

In a portion of the study reported by Durieux-Smith and associates (1985), repeat Crib-o-gram tests were administered and low interscreen correlation coefficients were obtained (0.36 and 0.52 for preterm and older infants, respectively). Such correlations may have limited value, because scalar scores are probability estimates and not absolute values with a reference point.

High false-positive rates obtained with Crib-o-gram screening have been reported by Durieux-Smith and associates (1985) and Wright and Rabak (1983). These rates differ greatly from those obtained in the original validation studies with Crib-o-gram. A possible explanation for the high false-positive rates may lie in the calibration of the instruments. The microprocessor can only score digitized input waveforms that it assumes are accurate representations of neonatal motion. Further, the analyzer accepts for trial baseline motion that is within limits and is a function of transducer sensitivity, mattress thickness, bassinet angulation, and system gain. If any of these four factors vary significantly, the microprocessor does not recognize the "true" acceptable behavioral state of the infant and administers stimuli at a time when the likelihood of eliciting a response is minimal. This in turn leads to a higher than expected failure rate and false-positive error. Based on experience with many hospital sites when false-positive error rates exceed 14 percent for a large enough sample, there is a possibility that the Crib-o-gram may have been out of calibration.

Historically, there has been no means by which the Crib-o-gram operator can ascertain system function other than by trending screening results over prolonged periods of time. To solve this problem, a means of testing and calibrating the transducer and associated circuitry would be helpful. This type of calibration, then, would help to avoid the collection of data confounded with out-of-specification Crib-o-gram operation.

An advantage of the Crib-o-gram is its automatically defining the trial and delivering the acoustic stimulus. If future improvements included filtered waveforms recorded on an abbreviated strip chart, professionals could read "clean" waveforms, have a feedback mechanism for calibrating the system, have a comparison scoring (scalar) for validation, and have a permanent record of screening.

The Crib-o-gram has been successfully used in many screening programs. In order for Crib-o-gram screening to be effective, the screening staff (neonatologists, pediatricians, nurses, social workers, and audiologists) must work in concert to provide aggressive medical and audiological follow-up. An early diagnosis is the objective of screening so that educational or therapeutic intervention strategies or both can be executed.

REFERENCES

Burney, P., Mauldin, L., and Crump, B. (1974). Predicting hearing loss from the acoustic reflex. *Journal of Speech and Hearing Disorders, 39,* 11–22.

Downs, M. (1978, Fall). That a child may hear. *Deaf Research Foundation Record,* p. 1.

Downs, M. P., and Hemenway, W. G. (1969). Report on the hearing screening of 17,000 neonates. *International Audiology, 8,* 72–76.

Durieux-Smith, A., Picton, T., Edwards, C. G., Goodman, T. T., and MacMurray, B. (1985). The crib-o-gram in the NICU: An evaluation based in brainstem electric response audiometry. *Ear and Hearing, 6*(1), 20–24.

Feinmesser, M. (1976). Neonatal screening for detection of deafness. *Archives of Otolaryngology, 102,* 297–299.

Galambos, C., and Galambos, R. (1979). Brainstem evoked response audiometry in newborn hearing screening. *Archives of Otolaryngology, 105,* 86–90.

Gerber, S. E. (1977). Newborn and diagnostic screening tests. In B. F. Jaffe (Ed.), *Hearing loss in children* (pp. 78–88). Baltimore: University Park Press.

Keith, R. W. (1973). Impedance audiometry with neonates. *Archives of Otolaryngology, 97,* 465–467.

Luterman, D. M., and Chasin, J. (1970). The pediatrician and the parents of the deaf child. *Pediatrics, 45,* 115–116.

Miller, K., and Simmons, F. B. (1984). A retrospective and an update on the Crib-o-gram neonatal hearing screening audiometer. *Seminars in Hearing, 5*(1), 49–55.

Northern, J. L., and Downs, M. P. (1974). *Hearing in children.* Baltimore: Williams and Wilkins.

Ruben, R. J. (1978, May). Delay in diagnosis. *Volta Review,* pp. 201–202.

Shaw, C. P., Chandler, D., and Dale, R. (1978, May). Delay in referral of children with impaired hearing. *Volta Review,* pp. 206–215.

Simmons, F. B. (1977). Automated screening test for newborns: The Crib-o-gram. In B. F. Jaffe (Ed.), *Hearing loss in children.* Baltimore: University Park Press.

Simmons, F. B., McFarland, W. H., and Jones, F. R. (1979). An automated hearing screening technique for newborns. *Acta Otolaryngology, 87,* 1–8.

Simmons, F. B., and Russ, F. W. (1974). Automated newborn hearing screening, the Crib-o-gram. *Archives of Otolaryngology, 100,* 1–7.

Stein, L., Ozdamar, O., Kraus, N., and Paton, J. (1983). Follow-up of infants screened by auditory brainstem response in the neonatal intensive care unit. *Journal of Pediatrics, 103,* 447–453.

Wright, L. B., and Rabak, L. P. (1983). Crib-o-gram (COG) and ABR. Effect of variables on test results. *Journal of Acoustical Society of America* (Suppl. 1), *74,* 540.

Chapter **5**

The Auditory Brainstem Response in Neonatal Hearing Screening

John T. Jacobson
Martyn L. Hyde

In preceding chapters, the focus has been on describing in detail the rationale and development of neonatal hearing screening programs. We have learned that a functional auditory system is a prerequisite for the acquisition of speech and language skills. An important aspect of these cognitive processes is a strategic developmental state that encompasses the first 2 years of life. Logic suggests that any auditory dysfunction within this period may significantly degrade basic learning experiences. Evolved from this premise has been an emphasis on early detection of hearing loss and the establishment of intervention programs and habilitative management. Previous experience indicates that mass infant screening, that is, the testing of every live birth, is impractical and not economically justifiable. The development of the high-risk register has offered a method of selectively categorizing an infant sub-population that is more susceptible to congenital or early-onset hearing impairment. The implementation of the register has allowed audiologists and other hearing health specialists to focus on procedural evaluation and development of techniques that have led to improved identification criteria and test efficiency.

Initially, behavioral observation audiometry (BOA) was used in newborn auditory screening programs as the sole basis for estimating hearing impairment. However, concern regarding the validity and repeatability of behavioral testing in this age group provided the impetus for the development of electrophysiological measures as a screening technique. Until the clinical implementation of the auditory brainstem response (ABR), no screening procedure had been available to provide a relatively objective assessment of auditory function in the newborn population. The ABR is currently an accepted tool in audiological and neurological assessment and is being used extensively with healthy babies and graduates of intensive care nurseries (ICN). With this in mind, the purpose of this chapter is to describe the strengths and limitations of the ABR as a tool for newborn hearing screening. The remainder of this section will be devoted to a brief overview of the events and rationale that have contributed to the current role of the ABR. In the next section, we will describe the normative properties of the ABR, emphasizing subject and stimulus variables. The final section will discuss ongoing programs and offer a perspective on current practice.

HISTORICAL DEVELOPMENT

Over the years, hearing practitioners involved in infant testing have been primarily concerned with behavioral techniques. Newborn screening with BOA uses visual observation of an infant's response to a particular auditory stimulus without reinforcement. Most behavioral screening protocols involve a test stimulus having a wideband frequency spectrum between 750 and 4000 Hz, peaking near 3000 Hz and presented in excess of 90 dB SPL. Response criteria are based on an "arousal response," which involves generalized body and simultaneous eye movement. The proper role of this type of behavioral newborn hearing screening is simply to rule out profound bilateral hearing loss. For infants, usually from 3 to 6 months of age, a form of operant conditioning is used to obtain the desired behavioral response. Observed infant responses are usually gauged against some expected degree of alerting and localization to the auditory stimulus in a sound field. The application of such a behavioral procedure for this age group remains suspect in light of the absence of adequate validating criteria and established norms. Recently, visual reinforcement audiometry (VRA) in infants has been shown to be a more promising tool for hearing assessment (Trehub, Schneider, and Bull, 1981; Wilson and Thompson, 1984). Despite its success, VRA has been restricted to infants 6 months through 2 years of age and is impractical as a hearing screening measure because of time and procedural complexities.

For the past two decades, behavioral screening in the newborn nursery was *the* accepted procedure. However, behavioral testing has come under a great deal of scrutiny due to the high rate of false positives and false negatives reported in the literature (Feinmesser and Tell, 1971; Feinmesser, Tell, and Levi, 1982; McFarland and Simmons, 1980; Northern and Downs, 1984; Parving, Elberling, and Salomon, 1981). In its most recent position statement, the Joint Committee on Infant Hearing (1982) rejected the universal use of auditory testing of all newborn infants but was not specific about what behavioral or electrophysiological methods are appropriate. Recently, three studies have compared behavioral and electrophysiological (ABR) newborn screening and have shown that the sensitivity and specificity of behavioral observation and automated behavioral (Crib-o-gram) hearing screening are suspect; the further use of such procedures in newborn testing is questioned (Durieux-Smith, Edwards, Picton and MacMurray, 1985; Durieux-Smith and Jacobson, 1985; Jacobson and Morehouse, 1984).

From the outset, it is important to recognize that the evolution of the ABR technique is itself in a state of infancy, particularly as it applies to the measurement of hearing sensitivity. During the mid-1970s, first reports began to surface that substantiated the use of ABR as an evaluation process in healthy and premature newborn infants (Hecox, 1975; Hecox and Galambos, 1974; Mokotoff, Schulman-Galambos, and Galambos, 1977; Salamy and McKean, 1976; Salamy, McKean, and Buda, 1975; Schulman-Galambos and Galambos, 1975; Starr, Amlie, Martin, and Sanders, 1977). These investigations established the basic features of threshold measurement, input-output function (e.g., intensity-latency, intensity-amplitude), maturational change, and age-dependent norms. Most important was the successful demonstration of an objective electrophysiological procedure capable of detecting transient and permanent hearing loss in newborns and infants. Furthermore, the ABR provided insight into the pathophysiology of auditory and neurological deficits and has been used in conjunction with radiological and otological evidence.

The first application of the ABR as a hearing screening procedure can be traced to an International Conference on Early Diagnosis of Hearing Loss (Gerber and Mencher, 1978). The conference focused on procedures and techniques that would detect, confirm, and quantify hearing loss within the first 6 months of life. Generated from this conference was a series of resolutions that centered on identifying procedures; two recommendations were germane to auditory evoked potentials and their use with infants and children. The first resolution encouraged the use of electric response audiometry (ERA)—a generic term covering many types of evoked potential procedures in the audiological test battery for children, and the second resolution urged further research into ABR audiometry in the newborn ICN. The latter resolution acknowledged the growth and impact ABR methods would have in the newborn nursery environment. Specific to the test procedure, it was recommended that the following information be gathered and incorporated into a screening report:

1. Latency of ABR wave V response as a function of the click intensity
2. Threshold estimates
3. Statement of the type of hearing loss found, if any
4. Measurement of the I–V interval of the ABR

It was at this conference that Galambos (1978) presented the first working model for the assessment of infants suspected of having hearing loss. The model was predicated on ABR infant testing within the first 2 months of life. An infant was considered to have failed the test if a replicable wave V response was not present in either ear at 30 dB HL, given age corrected latency values based on established norms. Subsequently, Schulman-Galambos and Galambos (1979) reported ABR results on 220 normal and 75 ICN babies as part of a routine neonatal hearing screening program and on 325 additional ICN babies who were 1 year of age or older. Two important findings emerged from their study: First, the ABR was determined to be a viable screening tool in the ICN; second, when both ICN groups were coalesced, totaling 373 high-risk infants, 1 in 47 (2.1 percent) showed severe hearing deficits in at least one ear. The incidence of hearing loss in intensive care graduates and other infants at risk for hearing loss is significantly greater than in the total infant population (1 in 1000; Carrel, 1977), and this finding has been substantiated in subsequent investigations.

Is the ABR the solution to behavioral newborn hearing screening? Certainly a wealth of information attesting to its value in the newborn and infant is mounting. With few exceptions (Cox, Hack, and Metz, 1982; Downs, 1982; Roberts et al., 1982), ABR methods have become widely accepted as a hearing screening tool in the newborn nursery. Galambos, Hicks, and Wilson (1984) claim that the ABR offers high test efficiency and reliability and is a relatively cost-effective means of infant hearing screening. Some advantages and limitations of ABR procedures are discussed in a later section.

ABR PROPERTIES AND MEASUREMENTS

Despite the endorsements found in the literature, there are many technical, procedural, physiological, and pathological variables that may act either independently or in concert to affect response measurement. Although the validity and reliability of ABR measures have been fairly well established for adult subjects, some evidence has questioned the reliability of ABR as a screening measure in the pediatric age group and, in particular, with high-risk infants (Cox, Hack, and Metz, 1981a; Salamy, 1984; Salamy, Mendelson, Tooley, and Chaplin, 1980). Given that variability of response parameters is inherent in the signal-to-noise problem and that maturation has a significant effect on the infant ABR, it is vital that every effort be made to identify and control sources of error in ABR measurement and interpretation. Only in this manner can baseline information be confidently collected to form a data pool by which abnormal response measurement can be defined. The remainder of this section addresses some important aspects of variability that affect infant brainstem response measurement and interpretation.

RESPONSE FEATURES AND CRITERIA

At high stimulus intensity levels, the first detectable brainstem response traces can be observed as early as the 28th gestational week in the premature newborn (Starr et al., 1977; Stockard, Stockard, and Coen, 1983). Recently, Galambos and associates (1984) reported ABR results on 2900 newborn ears and showed that by the 30th week, 83 percent generated ABRs and 30 dB clicks in either one or both ears. By term (40th week), 91 percent responded to low levels of click stimulus.

The newborn brainstem response produced by click stimulation consists of three major vertex- or forehead-positive peaks equivalent to waves I, III, and V in the adult. Waves II and IV emerge later in development, but by 1 year of age, the morphology of an infant response resembles that of the adult.

There are two distinct but interrelated applications that may be incorporated into ABR assessment. The first involves the status and sensitivity of the peripheral hearing mechanism, including the middle ear and cochlea, whereas the second relates to the neural integrity of the acoustic nerve and caudal regions of the brainstem pathway.

The primary goal of our screening test is to rule out congenital or very early-onset hearing loss. The presence or absence of a particular response component will serve as a measure of pass or fail. For example, let us assume that a response at 30 dB normal hearing level (nHL) has been defined as a passing screening intensity. Those infants who produce a replicable wave component pass the screen; those who show no response fail the test. For these purposes, the presence or absence of a brainstem response may be considered the predictive measure. Usually, the wave V component is selected because it is prominent and detectable at low sensation levels.

The choice of pass-fail intensity criterion will directly affect the operating characteristics of any screening procedure. As the criterion intensity level is lowered, more hearing-impaired babies will fail; the sensitivity of the test will improve, but the false-positive rate increases. In contrast, if a higher intensity is selected (e.g., 40 or 50 dB nHL), the false-negative rate will increase because more abnormal infants will pass the test, but the false-positive rate (those normal hearing babies who failed the test) will decrease. For a detailed account of the operating characteristics of a screening test see Chapter 2 of this text.

Auditory screening with the ABR often includes consideration of response component latency and amplitude. Figure 5–1 illustrates the various latency and amplitude measurement characteristics from a brainstem response. The absolute latency of a vertex-positive wave is normally measured in milliseconds (msec) from the stimulus onset to some point on the wave peak, usually immediately prior to the negative slope of the wave. Often, at high intensity levels, waves IV and V will converge, resulting in a broad wave with a bulge or shoulder on its negative slope. This point is frequently chosen as the latency of wave V. As in adults, the latency of waves III and V and, to a lesser degree, wave I decrease as intensity increases.

A second latency measure commonly used in the neurological aspects of the assessment is the interwave interval (IWI) or interpeak (IPL). This measure reflects the latency difference between two peak components and is considered to reflect the neural conduction time between physiological generators within the eighth nerve and brainstem pathway. The IWI has been used in the demonstration of perinatal asphyxia; infectious diseases, including bacterial meningitis and brainstem glioma; intracranial hemorrhage; and neurodegenerative disorders such as Wilson's disease. In addition to prolonged IWIs, neurological abnormalities have also been characterized by reductions in the V/I amplitude ratio (<0.5), unusual response change to increases in stimulus repetition rate, and significant differences between ears in wave latency, given comparable peripheral sensitivity. A change in any one of these criteria may make an infant neurologically suspect and warrant further neurological, radiological, and audiological investigation. Table 5–1 presents the absolute latencies of waves I and V and the IWI of I–V for term infants from published studies.

In newborn screening, given normal neurological status, cochlear pathology will affect wave latency differentially. For cochlear hearing loss in the 1000 to 4000 Hz region, a delay in wave V latency is expected at moderate and low intensities. At higher intensity levels, wave V may be within normal latency limits. In contrast, conductive pathology will tend to prolong all wave latencies. A prolongation of

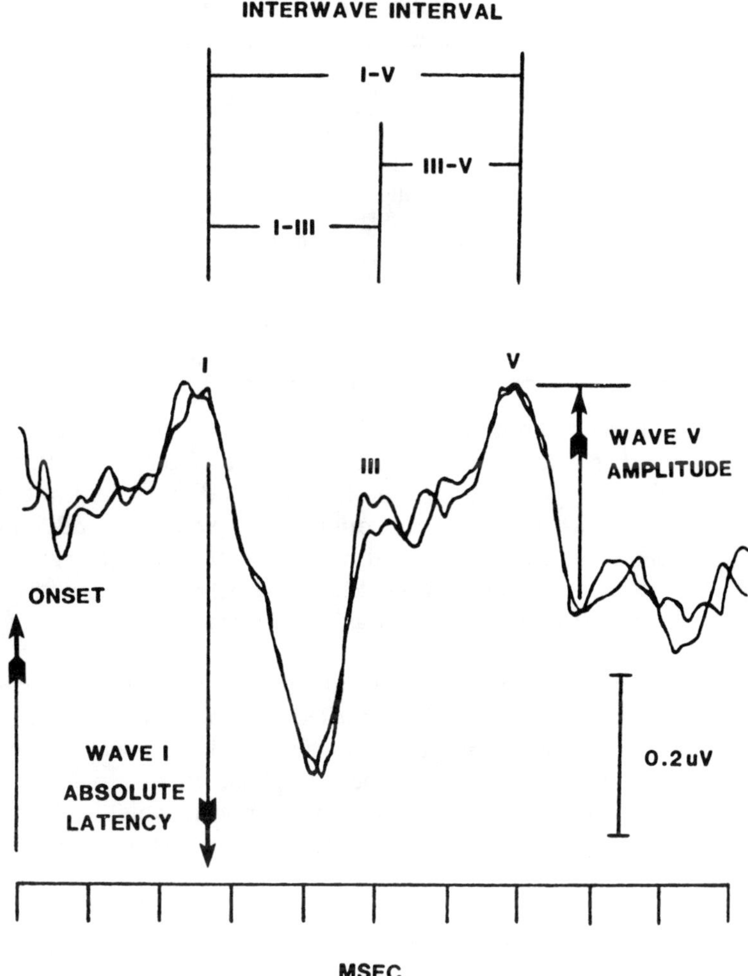

Figure 5–1. Newborn auditory brainstem response illustrating the latency, amplitude, and interwave interval measurement characteristics. Each trace represents the sum of 2000 trials.

the absolute latency of wave I is usually indicative of transient or permanent middle ear disorders, given a normal I–V latency interval.

The amplitude of a brainstem response is normally calculated in microvolts (μV) or nanovolts (nV) between two points, one of which is always the positive wave peak. The other point may be measured from the voltage baseline or the negative trough succeeding the peak. In adults, absolute amplitude tends to decrease differently as intensity decreases (Hecox and Galambos, 1974; Jewett, Romano, and Williston, 1970; Picton, Stapells, and Campbell, 1981).

Table 5–1. The Absolute and Relative ABR Latencies for Term Infants

			Wave		
Study	Click Intensity	Rate (seconds)	I	V	I–V
Starr et al. (1977)	65 dB HL	10/s	2.1	7.0	4.9
Despland and Galambos (1980)	60 dB HL	10/s	2.2	7.2	5.0
Galambos et al. (1982)	60 dB HL	10/s	2.2	7.2	5.0
Stockard and Stockard (1981)	60 dB HL	10/s	2.1	6.9	4.8
Finitzo-Hieber (1982)	60 dB HL	30/s	2.5	7.6	5.1
Jacobson et al. (1982)	60 dB HL	10/s	2.2	7.1	4.9
Salamy (1984)	60 dB HL	10/s	2.1	7.2	5.1
Cevette (1984)	60 dB HL	33/s	2.4	7.4	4.9
Cox (1985)	60 dB HL	10/s	2.3	7.1	4.7
Durieux-Smith et al. (1985)	70 dB HL	11/s	2.0	6.9	5.0

Unfortunately, in both adults and infants absolute amplitude can rarely be used as a diagnostic indicator, due to its inter- and intrasubject variability. Response amplitude is influenced by biological characteristics such as wave source orientation, volume conduction, tissue impedance properties, and neural synchrony (Hecox and Burkhard, 1982). As an alternative, Starr and Achor (1975) suggested the use of the V/I amplitude ratio as a more stable diagnostic measure.

Hecox and Cone (1981) have used the amplitude ratio successfully with high-risk infants. They studied 126 babies with acute episodes of asphyxia and reported that the amplitude ratio was a reliable predictor of longitudinal neurological sequelae in this risk group. Whether amplitude ratios will play a significant role in hearing screening remains unanswered, and more research is needed.

MATURATIONAL TRENDS

Maturational changes strongly influence the quantitative and qualitative analysis of infant ABRs. Figure 5–2 shows a series of ABRs from term to adulthood, illustrating characteristic maturational response changes. Typically, latency decreases while amplitude increases as a function of age. However, it is important to recall that individual ABR waves are affected differentially; this premise holds true for all waves, and the more rostral the response, the longer the developmental time course (Hecox and Burkhard, 1982).

Recently, Eggermont (1983) and Fria and Doyle (1984) have shown that two exponential curves having differing slope functions can be used to describe wave latency maturation. One curve with a steep function represents rapid maturation and is completed by the 50th week post-conception; a second more gradual curve reflects a

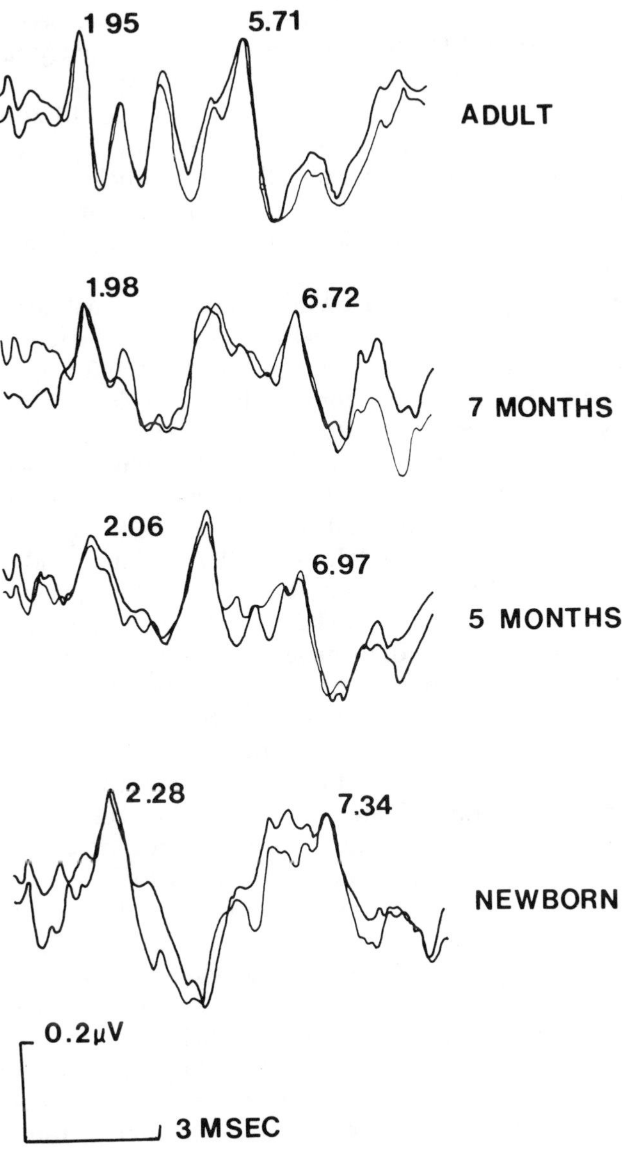

Figure 5–2. The effects of age on the auditory brainstem response. Note with increasing age the emergence of additional wave components and the reduction in wave latency. ABR traces resulted from 60 dB nHL monaural click stimuli presented at a rate of 10 per second. Forehead/vertex positivity is plotted upward in this and all subsequent figures.

slower maturational process ending by about 2 years of age. Waves I, III, and V all show a similar rapid maturation initially, whereas the latter two waves are characterized by an additional second lower curve slope. Fria and Doyle also calculated wave latency ratios as a function of age and showed that all ratios were independent of age during the first stage of maturation, whereas waves III and V were independent of age during the second stage. They suggested that in view of similar wave functions for all waves initially, peripheral as well as central changes contribute to latency maturation. Further, they suggested that latency ratios could be used to estimate hearing loss in newborns.

At term, the latency of wave V for a healthy normal-hearing newborn is about 7.1 in response to a 60 dB nHL click. The rate of latency shift of wave V in premature infants is about 0.2 to 0.3 ms per week as gestational age increases from 30 to 40 weeks (Despland and Galambos, 1980; Hecox and Burkhard, 1982). As noted, wave V latency decreases nonlinearly until 24 months, when it reaches adult value (Hecox and Galambos, 1974; Salamy and McKean, 1976), whereas wave I approaches adult latency by the third month of life (Jacobson, Morehouse, and Johnson, 1982; Salamy and McKean, 1976). These differential changes that occur in the peripheral and central auditory mechanism have been attributed to improved middle ear transmission, improved cochlear and acoustic nerve sensitivity, and changes in myelination and synaptic efficiency.

Because of differential wave latency effects, the IWI is also age dependent. At term, the I–V interval for a newborn is about 5.0 ms for a click stimulus. According to Salamy (1984), the developmental trends for IWI I–V and I–III are similar from 33 weeks PCA onward, thus reflecting the slower maturation of the more rostral brainstem responses. These changes in latency are shown in Figure 5–3. Note the decrease in latency for waves I and V and the I–V interwave interval over time.

The trend of shorter absolute and relative latencies found in female adults (Jacobson, Novotny, and Elliott, 1980; McClelland and McCrea, 1979) is not evident in healthy newborns. Stockard, Stockard, Westmoreland, and Corfits (1979) found no statistical differences in relative latency measures in 77 normal term babies. Durieux-Smith and associates (1985) studied 434 newborns ranging from 32 to 56 weeks gestational age and found no difference between male and female babies for either response amplitude or latency. Jacobson and colleagues (1982) also found no difference in amplitude or latency measures in 124 newborns between 40 and 50 weeks gestational age and suggested that response values could be coalesced for clinical manipulation without statistical variance. In contrast, others (Cox, Hack, and Metz, 1981b; Pauwels, Vogeleer, Clements, Rousseeuw,

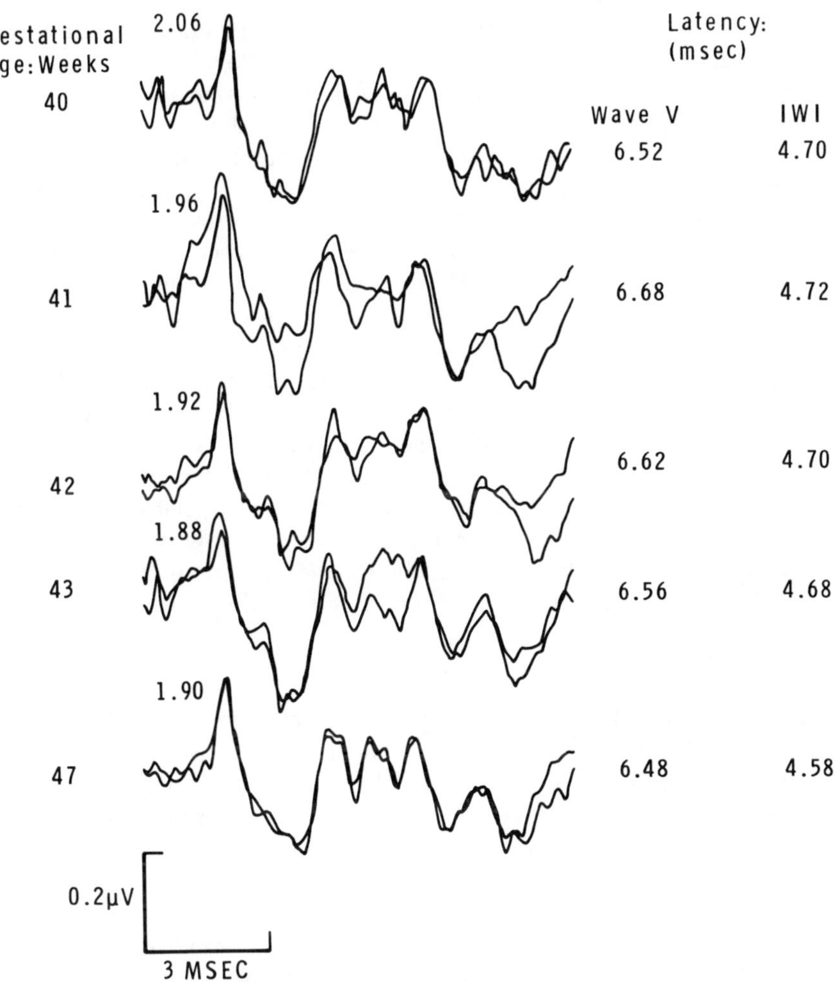

Figure 5–3. Serial auditory brainstem responses from one newborn over a 2-month period. Note decreased absolute and relative latencies as a function of increasing age. Each trace represents a total of 2000 click stimuli presented monaurally at 60 dB nHL at a rate of 10 per second.

and Kaufman, 1982) have reported latency differences in premature infants. These differences may be more related to the neurological status of premature newborns than to gender effects.

STIMULUS PARAMETERS

To date, the click stimulus has been used almost exclusively with ABR newborn screening. Although stimulus polarity may vary (see

Polarity in this section), unfiltered clicks are generated by driving a transducer (earphone) with a rectangular voltage pulse of approximately 100 μsec duration. Because of their near-instantaneous onset, they are capable of initiating more synchronized neural excitation and of producing a more defined ABR than other stimuli with longer onset-offset envelopes. The click stimulus has consistently elicited clear brainstem responses at low intensities corresponding to levels near adult behavioral threshold. There are, however, recognized limitations when using clicks (Hyde, 1985). Due to their wide energy-density spectrum, the click tends to initiate extensive activity of a large number of auditory neurons, thereby eliminating any frequency specificity. Therefore, the click-generated ABR must be considered a representation of the mid to high (1000–4000+ Hz) frequency range. Hearing sensitivity beyond these frequency limits is unquantifiable by click stimuli. As a consequence, click stimulus screening programs are restricted in their analysis of newborn hearing status to a limited frequency range with no information regarding low-frequency residual hearing. With this in mind, the following comments will address click stimulus properties and their affects on the infant ABR.

Intensity

Stimulus attenuation will prolong wave latency in adults and infants. An example of such an intensity–latency (I–L) shift is illustrated for a newborn and normal hearing adult in Figure 5-4. The slope of the wave V I–L function has been reported to be age-dependent and shallower than that found in adults (Despland and Galambos, 1980; Hecox, 1975; Jacobson et al., 1982). Figure 5-5 demonstrates this slope difference. Latency values presented in Figure 5-4 have been plotted into an I–L function. The wave V latency shift increases in newborns at a rate of approximately 35 μsec per dB (Hecox and Galambos, 1974; Jacobson et al., 1982; Schulman-Galambos and Galambos, 1975).

The rate of wave I latency shift with intensity has been reported approximately equal to that of wave V by some investigators (Jacobson et al., 1982; Salamy, 1984), and greater by other investigators (Cox, 1985; Stockard et al., 1979). These reported differences are important relative to the I–V interwave interval in newborns. If the absolute I–L shifts are similar, the IWI will remain intensity-independent; however, if differences exist, the IWI will decrease with decreasing intensity. Regardless of these reported differences, a 60 dB nHL click stimulus will produce a I–V latency interval of about 5.0 msec in newborns.

The amplitude of waves I and V in newborns has also been shown to decrease with a reduction in intensity, whereas wave III

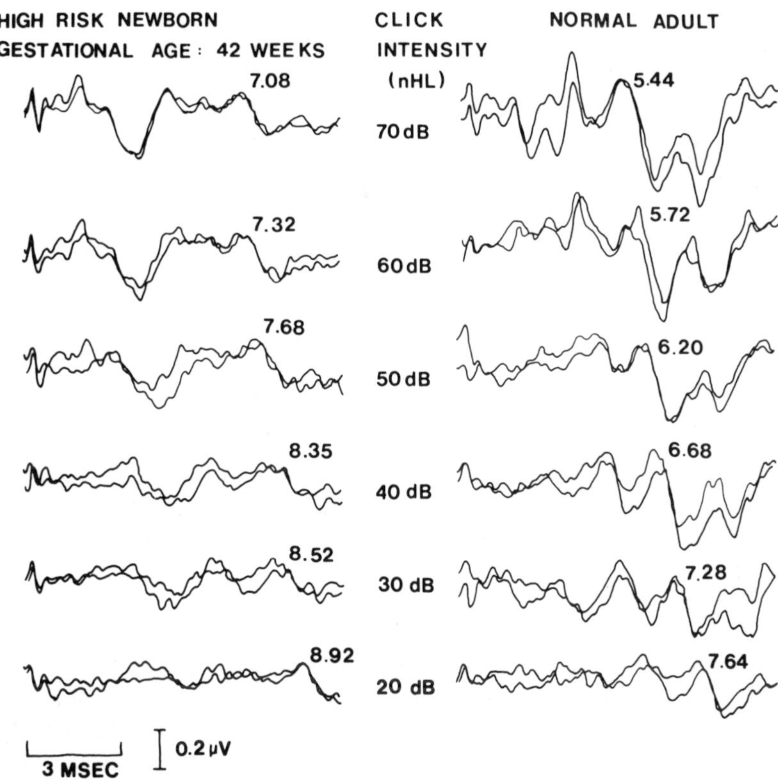

Figure 5–4. A series of auditory brainstem responses with decreasing intensity. Each trace represents the sum of 2000 click stimuli presented monaurally to a newborn and adult at a rate of 10 per second.

remains relatively stable. In contrast, amplitude will increase as a function of age, reaching asymptote at approximately 2 to 4 years (Durieux-Smith et al., 1985; Jacobson et al., 1982; Salamy, 1984). The amplitude of a newborn wave I response is about double that of wave V (Jacobson et al., 1982; Salamy and McKean, 1977; Starr et al., 1977).

The adult V/I amplitude ratio consistently exceeds 2.0 (Stockard, Stockard, and Sharbrough, 1978). However, there is some disagreement as to the ratio expected in newborns. Gafni, Sohmer, Gross, Weizman, and Robinson (1980) and Jacobson and associates (1982) reported values less than 1.0, whereas other investigators have shown values slightly in excess of 1.0 (Durieux-Smith et al., 1985; Hecox and Burkhard, 1982; Salamy, 1984). These minor differences may be attributed to measurement technique and not to physiological

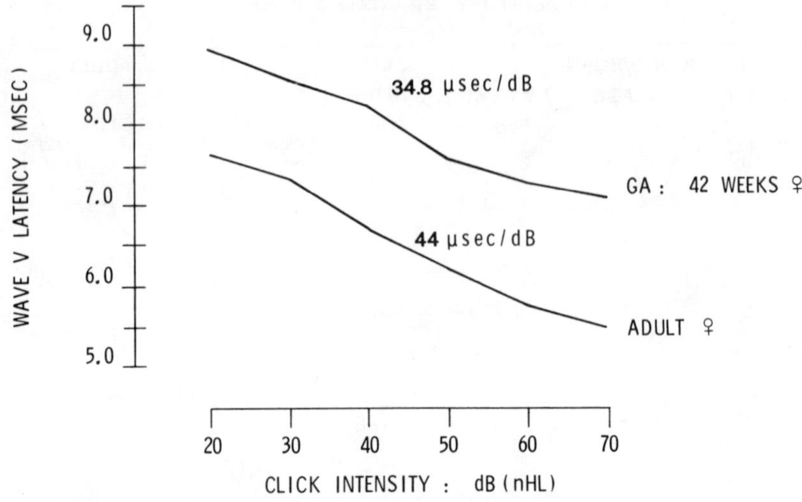

Figure 5–5. Plotted intensity–latency curve functions for brainstem responses obtained in Figure 5–4. Major slope differences exist between newborn and adult responses.

dependencies. The amplitude ratio is affected by stimulus intensity and repetition rate and is shown to increase until age 2 years, when it reaches adult value (Hecox and Jacobson, 1984; Jacobson et al., 1982; Salamy, Fenn, and Bronshvag, 1979; Stockard et al., 1978). The V/I amplitude ratio is plotted in Figure 5–6 and depicts age-related dependencies.

Rate

A change in stimulus repetition rate will affect latency, amplitude, and wave morphology in infants and adults. An increase in rate tends to increase wave latency, with corresponding decreases in amplitude (Salamy, McKean, Pettett, and Mendelson, 1978; Stockard et al., 1979). Rate effects have been measured in premature infants as early as the 32nd week post-conception to click stimuli at rates of up to 80 per second (Despland and Galambos, 1980). At rates less than 10 per second, negligible changes should be anticipated.

Rate effects have been shown to interact linearly with intensity (Hecox and Burkhard, 1982) and age (Durieux-Smith et al., 1985). The largest latency shift is seen from wave V, which increases at a rate of 0.014 msec per Hz in infants. Infants younger than 8 months of age produce a wave V shift of about 1 msec for a 70 per second rate increase, whereas wave I will shift by 0.4 msec. These differences will

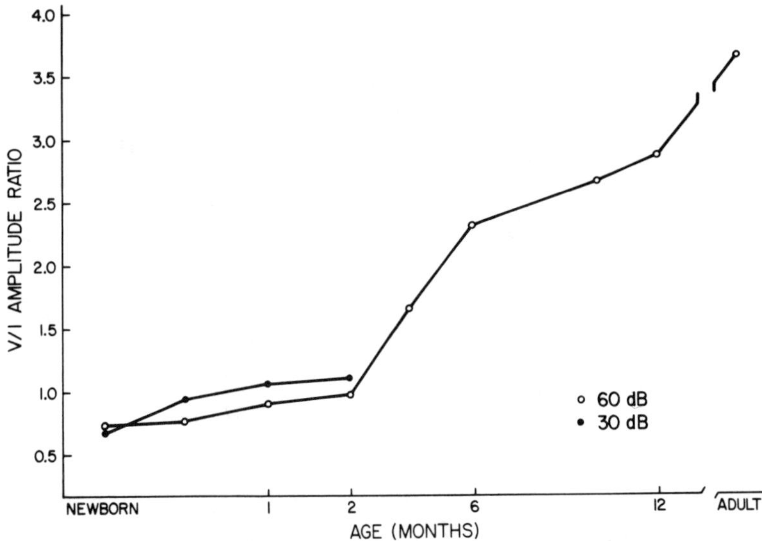

Figure 5–6. The V/I auditory brainstem response amplitude ratio. The amplitude ratio is plotted for two intensities from term to 2 months and 60 dB nHL from 2 months onward.

result in a rate-related increase in the I–V IWI. The interaction of rate and age have also been noted. Durieux-Smith and associates (1985) reported latency shifts of 1.3 msec between 11 and 61 per second in 30-week gestational age prematures and a shift of 0.6 msec for 56-week-old newborns, exhibiting an average slope of 38 μsec per week. Thus, normative data must take into account both intensity and age when various rates of stimulus presentation are applied in the screening process.

Wave amplitudes are also affected differentially by rate change; generally, as rate increases, wave amplitudes are diminished. Recently, Durieux-Smith and associates (1985) found that the amplitudes of waves I and V significantly decreased with rate increases, whereas wave III remained stable. Increases in repetition rate and long-term continuous stimulation have shown no evidence of habituation (Salamy and McKean, 1977), fatigue (Schulman-Galambos and Galambos, 1975), or refractoriness (Salamy, 1984) in the infant population. Because the amount of averaging per unit of time increases with increasing rate and because rates up to 40 per second have little effect on wave morphology, higher repetition rates may be more efficient. The effects of rate change on latency and amplitude are presented in Figure 6–7. Brainstem responses are from a newborn at 10 and 80 per second using a constant intensity of 60 dB nHL.

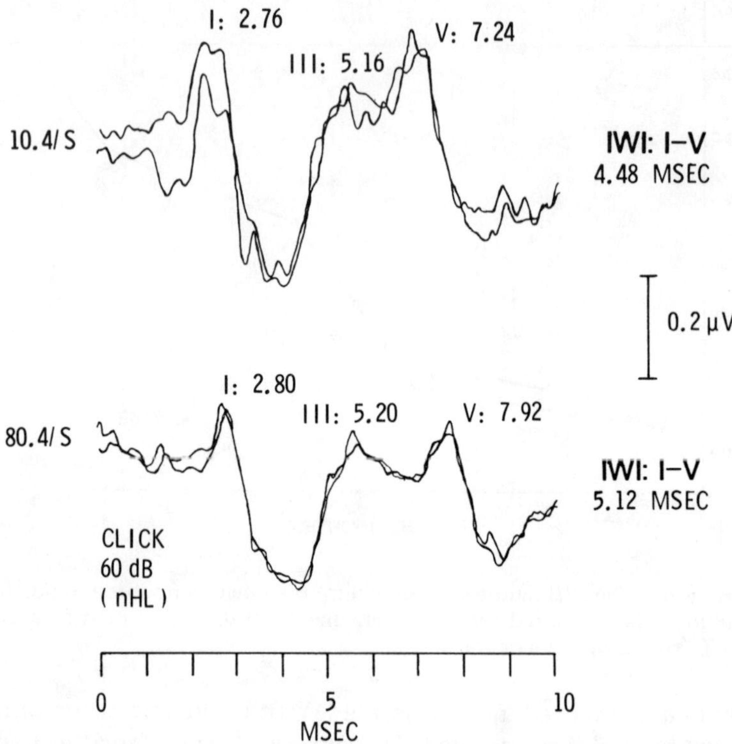

Figure 5–7. The effects of rate on an infant auditory brainstem response. Note the prolongation of absolute and relative latencies as rate increases. Each trace represents the sum of 2000 trials presented at 60 dB nHL.

Polarity

The initial direction of motion of a transducer is determined by the electrical polarity of the driving voltage pulse. A stimulus such as a click may be presented with a constant initial polarity or alternating polarity. Cann and Knott (1979) reported the problems associated with polarity measurement, and it appears that describing the acoustic profile of the tympanic membrane rather than the electric drive to the transducer is less problematic. Condensation or positive pressure will move the eardrum in an inward direction, whereas initial negative pressure or outward movement of the eardrum is caused by a rarefaction stimulus.

The excitation of primary auditory neurons is thought to occur only with basilar membrane movement generated by rarefaction polarity (Kiang, Watanabe, Thomas, and Clark, 1965). Hence, signal polarity may influence wave morphology and latency (Picton et al.,

1981; Stockard et al., 1979). Generally, earlier wave components are more affected, and wave I has shown consistently shorter latencies to rarefaction stimuli (Coats and Martin, 1977; Stockard et al., 1978). Stockard and colleagues (1979) reported prolonged neural conduction in newborns using rarefaction clicks. The literature is sparse concerning signal polarity effects and infant testing. In adults, the literature is conflicting. In the authors' opinion, significant advantages of one polarity over another have not been demonstrated conclusively. Alternating polarity might result in unpredictable summation effects on ABR morphology, and the need to check for this in cases of abnormal brainstem responses must be weighed against the convenience of stimulus artifact suppression.

Electrode Placement

In the averaging process, brainstem responses are volume conducted from subcortical levels and extracted from spontaneous electrical activity. Electroencephalographic (EEG) activity is commonly monitored using surface disk or cup electrodes. In order to provide gain and to improve the signal-to-noise ratio, electrodes are connected to a differential preamplifier. These devices require a minimum input of three electrodes. Several designations have been given to these electrodes, but the terms *inverting, noninverting,* and *common* describe their action most explicitly.

The role of the differential preamplifier is to amplify the *difference* in neural activity between the noninverting and inverting electrodes. In essence, electrical activity common to these two electrodes is almost totally eliminated, leaving only the difference. Electrode placement can affect ABR waveform. Thus, the correct positioning of electrodes is essential in the ABR screening process.

In the pediatric age group, a three-electrode montage is most frequently used. Usually the noninverting electrode is attached to the vertex (C_z) or forehead (F_z), and the inverting electrode is placed on the mastoid (Mi) or earlobe (Ai) of the stimulated ear. The common electrode is placed contralaterally. This vertical montage will enhance the amplitude of wave V, whereas a horizontal (earlobe to earlobe) montage has been reported to produce a more robust wave I in 70 percent of infants younger than 8 months of age (Hecox and Burkhard, 1982).

Band-Pass Filtering of the EEG

The band-pass EEG filter is an important component of the ABR recording system, because it can affect both response detectability and morphology. Detectability influences threshold, and morphology influences such features as absolute and relative latency and amplitude parameters. The variation between laboratories of filter types, cut-off frequencies, and slopes is a significant source of difficulty when comparing norms. In adult otoneurological ABR applications, the effects of both analog and digital filters are quite well known (e.g., Doyle and Hyde, 1981). In infants, we can expect similar filter effects on suprathreshold ABR morphology. A detailed discussion of these effects is not possible here; however, the important points are that filters can change amplitudes and latencies drastically and that these effects must be kept in mind when reading published reports or when relating experimental findings to the work of others.

In threshold estimation with the ABR, the effects of filter parameters have not been studied in depth. The problem is to optimize the detectability of the ABR, and this involves different considerations than those that are relevant to otoneurological assessment. As stimulus intensity is reduced, the energy spectrum of the ABR moves apically. It is the ABR spectrum near threshold that is relevant to filter optimization for detectability purposes. The high-pass filter segment will be the most influential, not only because the EEG noise level (mostly electromyogenic) is greatest at low frequency but also because this filter component will have the most marked effect on ABR morphology as a result of phase distortion.

For tonepip ABR recording, the near-threshold ABR morphology is totally unlike that of the classic moderate-intensity click ABR (Hyde, 1985). Certainly, if low-frequency tonepip ABRs are recorded with high-pass filter settings that are appropriate for neurological click ABR measures, thresholds will be elevated because of loss of ABR amplitude. Also, whereas phase distortion is undesirable in otoneurological recordings, it may actually be advantageous in threshold measurement, because the change in response waveform may make it more detectable. Further research is needed for optimization of filter conditions for ABR threshold measurement; for the moment, recommendations in the literature should be viewed with caution.

This section describing normative properties and the variables that influence their behavior may indeed seem formidable. Our intent is to point out that ABR testing is more than purchasing a clinical averager, plugging it in, testing a patient, and somehow estimating auditory sensitivity. Validity is the key to any new clinical technique, and the establishment of a normative data base is the first precursor in auditory assessment. The selection of stimulus parameters, the control of procedural variables, and the knowledge of maturational effects will reduce the chance of test error. These factors can, through careful and often time-consuming effort, be overcome, but they cannot be dismissed.

A PERSPECTIVE ON CURRENT PRACTICES

The general goals of early hearing assessment programs are to detect, quantify, and characterize significant hearing loss in order to facilitate prompt and appropriate management. In essence, the Joint Committee Position Statement recommends that by 6 months of age, the processes of detecting hearing loss and of describing it in sufficient detail to provide a quantitative basis for habilitation should be well advanced. This must be contrasted with past and, in some areas, current situations in which detection does not occur until 2 years of age or more or in which *habilitation* is merely an extenuated process of hearing investigation. At present, there is little hard evidence indicating that early intervention is effective. Such evidence is extremely difficult to gather in a prospective manner, and retrospective studies are influenced by a host of confounding variables. Nevertheless, there is an increasing body of supporting data that suggests that many aspects of auditory and related performance could be compromised by delayed management. It is certainly appropriate that early hearing assessment programs be included in high-quality health care delivery systems. Thus, the Joint Committee recommendations are a desirable target.

In health care generally, a major consideration in screening program establishment is the follow-up system; there is little purpose in detecting a disease unless definite and effective steps can be taken to cure or ameliorate it. Thus, the follow-up resources must be sufficient to cope with the yield of the screening program. For the early hearing assessment process to be justifiable, it is essential that the necessary medical, audiological, and other health-related delivery systems are in place and prepared to act rapidly and concretely on the basis of test results. Where the major test is ABR based, it follows that concrete habilitative steps may have to be taken on the basis of ABR findings alone.

In order to achieve effectiveness and efficiency, a number of factors must be taken into account in early assessment program design. Some of the basic considerations are whom to test, when, and how. There are also the questions of relating test outcomes to recommendations and subsequent actions. Finally, the matter of cost-effectiveness requires quantitative understanding of program resource requirements, yield, and costs of omission or error. The remainder of this section addresses some of these issues based on our own experiences administering infant screening programs.

Whom to Test

Since it is impossible to test all babies, selection rules must be applied to determine who will receive ABR testing. Whatever selection procedure is adopted, it can itself be viewed as a *test*, and it will have its own performance characteristics (.e.g, sensitivity and specificity). No selection process is perfect. It is essential to note that the overall error performance of a series of *tests* will be dominated by the worst aspects of each component in the series; this is true for both false-positive and false-negative errors. As a simple example, even if the ABR screening test were totally error-free, a program that includes a prior selection procedure based on risk factors will result in failure to detect most hearing loss of recessive genetic origin. Recall that a high percentage of "acquired" sensory hearing loss detected in early childhood may be attributed to genetic factors unknown to family members. For this particular etiology, the sensitivity of the risk evaluation *test* is abysmal.

In spite of the limitations of selection by risk factors, that process is a necessity in view of finite health care resources. There is no alternative procedure with adequate performance characteristics. Thus, in most screening programs, the determination of risk is the first *test*. Overall performance will be affected not only by the true predictive value of each risk factor but also by the availability and quality of the information upon which the risk assessment is to be based. Risk cannot be assessed if the necessary *test* has not been performed, or if the risk factor has not been properly documented. Certainly, there are significant variations between centers and between patient groups within centers in terms of perinatal assessment practices and levels of documentation.

ICN graduates are a convenient and reasonable starting point for development of early assessment programs; many of these babies will have at least one of the Joint Committee risk factors, especially low birthweight and anoxia. Extending the risk evaluation to the General Nursery can be very resource consumptive, and, in this much larger group, familial hearing loss and ENT malformations are the main targets. The recessive nature of much familial impairment is a serious problem. The Joint Committee register is a good basis, but there is certainly a need for better quantification of factors and criterion levels in relation to auditory and neurological sequelae. A useful review of risk factors has been presented by Gerkin (1984). It should be noted that classical risk factors are biased toward severe sensory impairments that are identifiable at a later age when traditional perceptual test formats become acceptably valid. Yet, ABR-based programs are dealing with neonates and infants younger than 6 months of age, and there is increasing concern about the ability to quantify hearing losses that are mild or moderate, unilateral, frequency specific, and not exclusively sensory. When the spectrum of disease to be detected is extended, it is necessary to re-examine the risk criteria and their performance.

In some centers, all ICN graduates are considered to be at risk, whereas in other centers, a further filtering by the high-risk register is applied. The proportion of ICN babies who will be formally at risk will vary considerably between ICNs, which themselves vary greatly in terms of their intake criteria and population characteristics. Furthermore, in some centers the practice is to select cases for ABR testing not only on the basis of risk factors but also according to the outcome of some behavioral screening test, either conventional or automated. Here, the over-all chain of *test* might be ICN graduation—formal risk assessment—behavioral testing—ABR testing. Over-all errors will be dominated by the selection rules and by the inherent insensitivity and inaccuracy of most, if not all, behaviorally based indices.

When to Test

The major concerns here are test validity, error rates, relevance and practicality. Provided that the ABR is done with correct methodology, in a well baby, in an appropriate environment, there is little reason at present to suspect significant change in the inherent validity of the ABR as a threshold estimation tool over the period from term to 6 months of age. Of course, since there is no reference hearing test of sufficient accuracy to validate the ABR in that age range, the validity is based on indirect inference, such as the observations that most click ABR thresholds in non-risk babies are stable over time, are comparable to adult normal-hearing thresholds, and are in agreement with good behavioral data when the latter becomes sufficiently credible. However, persistent concerns about the validity of ABR-based hearing threshold estimates apply to babies with abnormal ABR morphology or with no ABR at the highest stimulus levels. Confounding of hearing tests by neurological immaturity or neuropathy is a strong possibility, especially in neonates. Another concern is the possible effect of incomplete development of cochlear function and place-frequency relationships.

Error in many ABR tests is dominated by EEG conditions and lack of methodological or interpretive skill. The extent to which myogenic EEG contamination can confound threshold estimation is not widely recognized. Assuming good EEG conditions and sufficient skill, direct threshold estimation (as opposed to indirect inference from latency functions, and so on) may be fairly accurate if the methodology is correct. Examples of common and serious methodological errors include (1) testing with unequal electrode impedances; (2) insufficient use of artifact rejection facilities; (3) insufficient replication; (4) use of inappropriate recording bandwidth; (5) failure to adapt strategies and criteria to the needs of the individual patient, especially with regard to EEG characteristics; and (6) failure to recognize collapse of the external meatus.

The matter of relevance of ABR results to subsequent management is quite complex. A major program design decision is whether to test before hospital discharge or on an outpatient basis before 6 months of age or both. Is a partitioning of the population into *normal* and *hearing impaired* on the basis of a test done before discharge relevant to the pattern of need for intervention and management that will exist at about 6 months of age? It all depends on the time course of hearing loss expression and development in the first few months of extrauterine life. Hearing loss that is not yet expressed cannot be detected, and hearing loss that is changing over time is difficult to quantify. Little is known about these matters. Classical epidemiological data concerning incidence of hearing loss largely reflect inferences from inaccurate methods of hearing assessment and are probably riddled with assumptions and errors. The current volume of ABR research will help to clarify the situation because the ABR is probably a better quantifier of hearing in the first few months of life than any other procedure currently available. In the interim, statements that indicate a specified percentage of childhood severe sensory hearing loss as congenital must be viewed with skepticism. With few etiological exceptions, such as radiologically verifiable cochlear agenesis, congenital expression of hearing loss is exceedingly difficult to verify. Congenital causes of hearing loss expressed subsequently are another matter.

The Joint Committee has recognized that certain risk factors may be associated with progressive hearing loss, and, in such cases, a neonatal test, and even a 6-month test, may be insufficient to detect emergent dysfunction. Patients with these risk factors must be followed periodically, even if ABR results are normal. The larger concern is that we are still unaware of the true extent of progressive hearing loss in the first few months of life. It follows that the false-negative rate of neonatal ABRs is open to question.

The other side of the coin is the possible resolution of hearing loss present neonatally and the potentially undesirable consequences of flagging a child as hearing impaired on the basis of transient dysfunction. Conductive disorders are the most common cause of this pattern, and the present limited ability to differentiate quantitatively between conductive and sensory hearing loss components, especially in neonates, compounds the problem. Acoustic immittance does not contribute greatly until the child is older than 6 months of age, and otoscopy is not considered definitive enough to initiate or withhold treatment in the first 3 or 4 months of life.

Middle-ear problems may coexist with sensory deficits, and even exclusively sensory disorders can clearly fluctuate in adults. It is, therefore, unwise to assume that in young infants sensory hearing loss is always either stable or progressive. It is feasible, for example, that maturation and neural plasticity might cause at least partial resolution of sensory deficits present neonatally.

It appears that until further research clarifies matters and unless there is a definite intention to intervene medically or audiologically in the first 3 months of life, there are potential drawbacks to neonatal ABR testing, primarily on grounds of relevance to habilitation and errors related to dynamic aspects of hearing loss. The true extent of these drawbacks has yet to be revealed.

Regardless of what is the theoretically optimal ABR test timing, more mundane and practical considerations may determine the actual events. Our experiences differ in this regard. The major argument put forward for neonatal ABR testing is that before discharge from the hospital, the baby is captive and, at least in theory, can be tested, whereas compliance with a request to return at 4 months may be low. In addition, one of us (JTJ) has found that it is easier to orchestrate testing before discharge. Others, such as Alberti, Hyde, Riko, Corbin, and Fitzhardinge (1985) have found it easier to schedule and administer testing on an outpatient basis. These differences suggest that the most practical route depends on local variables, including the size of population, program organization, physical resources, and so on. The question of compliance in follow-up testing is a subtle matter, and there are considerable differences in reported rates between centers. Socioeconomic and cultural factors seem to influence compliance, but the procedures adopted are probably most critical. It is desirable, for example, to establish rapport with the parent, to be persistent but accommodating, and to have the unqualified support of the child's physician. In spite of best efforts, contact may be lost or the parent may flatly refuse to bring the child for testing. In the latter case, the value of any testing is open to debate, because the parent is such an important element in habilitation.

Another practical factor that influences the timing of tests is the need for an adequate period of EEG free from myogenic interference in order to get useful ABR measures. ABR testing for threshold in babies who are not asleep is time consuming, requires great skills, and is potentially prone to serious error. Neonates sleep readily, but as the child approaches 6 months of age, sleep induction requires increasing patience, cunning, planning, and parental cooperation. If sedation is to be used routinely, the problem is usually (but not always) solved; however, medication complicates the issue, and not all practitioners are prepared to use it routinely. Also, the use of sedation presupposes that the testing is to be done in a setting in which there is adequate medical supervision and facilities.

Overall, although there may be some justification in test deferral until about 3 or 4 months of age, local conditions will determine the most appropriate practice in any particular center. Certainly, in high-risk infants, an ABR at any time is preferable to no ABR.

How to Test

The ABR testing methods are strongly determined by the goals and constraints of the early assessment program as a whole. First, it is essential to define the characteristics of the hearing losses that are to be detected and the characteristics that will trigger intervention. This may sound trite, but it is notable that many reports dealing with ABR screening do not deal explicitly with this aspect and its consequences. Hearing loss is not an all-or-none phenomenon; it is not entirely clear what constitutes ''normal'' hearing in a neonate or young infant, and both error patterns and yield will depend on the failure criteria. For a click ABR screen, for example, the yield of ''failure'' at 30 dB nHL may be double or triple that at 40 dB nHL (Hyde, Riko, Corbin, Moroso, and Alberti, 1984). If all failures are to receive some kind of follow-up such as ENT examination and further audiometry, there is a massive difference in the resource requirements for the two choices of screening criterion. Also, we must examine the clinical significance of detecting or missing cases for a given criterion and must take into account the possible effects of loading a follow-up system whose practitioners may be quite accustomed to acting on the basis of a novel and very sensitive screening test. There is little that is more damaging to the credibility of a new program or more frustrating for parents than to have the follow-up ''system'' pronounce much of the screening program yield as ''within normal limits.''

In the context of test methods, it is necessary to consider precisely what is meant by the term *screening test*, versus other terms such as *diagnostic* or *detailed* test. A feature of most so-called screening tests is that they are quick and easy to administer to large populations and they tend to be inexpensive, compared with some more definitive procedures. These requirements should not be translated to mean sloppy. Because a test is labeled a screening test, it does not follow that standards of instrumentation or of tester expertise can be lowered. Quite the opposite is true, since the screen is a critical step in the over-all delivery system. Thus, even the most basic ABR test is quite costly. It requires an appropriate instrument and test environment and a properly trained examiner. The instrument may cost $20,000 with a 5-year maintenance cost of $10,000. At 1000 tests per year, the equipment cost is $6 plus consumables, and to this we must add staff costs. The overall minimum cost is likely to exceed $20 per test. Because the majority of tests will be negative, the actual cost of identifying a hearing-impaired baby is much greater than this (Galambos et al., 1984).

The most basic ABR test on a neonate will take about 30 minutes. Much of this time is consumed in settling the baby and applying electrodes. On an outpatient basis, the time spent waiting for adequate periods of quiet EEG can be much greater. Because considerable time is spent in preparing the neonate for testing, it makes little sense to test at a single click intensity level, which would be in the true spirit of a screen. It takes roughly 1 minute to get an average ABR, provided that a sufficiently high stimulus repetition rate is used. Based on two ABR averages, it takes about 2 minutes to get a decision for a given stimulus condition. If the baby fails at the lowest intensity (e.g., 30 or 40 dB), it seems reasonable to proceed to at least one higher intensity (e.g., 60 or 70 dB) to get an indication of the severity of the problem. Using two ABR averages at two intensities for two ears, the total ABR measurement time would be about 8 to 10 minutes.

One might question the value of measurements at higher intensities, since a failure at the lower intensity will presumably indicate a more exhaustive follow-up ABR. It makes sense only to elaborate the testing if there is to be some differential action ensuing from the work, such as prioritization for the follow-up effort.

When testing infants on an outpatient basis at, for example, 3 months corrected age (i.e., 3 months after term or about 52 weeks PCA), the time and overhead costs in accessing and settling the baby are so large that the concept of a screening test has little meaning. The test will be elaborated (given good EEG conditions) until threshold estimates and neurological status have been fully explored. One might call such tests *diagnostic*, depending on one's definition of diagnosis. Can a specified dB level of hearing loss stand independent as a diagnosis? What is really meant by a 20, 50, or 70 dB hearing loss? Such semantic quibbles are secondary to the bottom line that we can draw a distinction between two types of ABR testing: that which examines one or two stimulus conditions per ear, and that which defines threshold precisely and explores the neurological status of the auditory brainstem pathways more fully.

As noted earlier in this chapter, the majority of ABR testing uses wideband stimuli such as the click. Some of the limitations of click testing for threshold estimation have been outlined by Hyde (1985), and the matter has been discussed in some depth by Stapells, Picton, Perez-Abalo, Reed, and Smith (1985). In particular, a normal click threshold may coexist with significant low-frequency or high-frequency hearing loss. The former might indicate clinically significant middle-ear dysfunction, and the latter might indicate progressive sensory impairment. If the click threshold is abnormal, frequency-specific assessment by ABR can reveal the audiometric contour and the amount of residual low-frequency hearing, both of which may influence management. Further research is needed to clarify the methods and clinical benefit of frequency-specific testing, which is generally more difficult and certainly more time consuming than click testing.

Another area of active research is that of differentiating conductive from cochlear impairment. The obvious method of direct bone conduction threshold estimation has difficulties associated with electrical artifact, coupling the transducer to the head, and transducer frequency response. Further research and development are likely to lead to viable bone-conduction procedures. In the interim, the practice of bone-conduction testing is not yet widespread, and we are usually obliged to attempt to infer the type of hearing loss from ABR latency functions. Undoubtedly, we can gather clues from such parameters as the latency of wave I and the slope of the wave V I–L function. Although there is little doubt that these features differ systematically between diagnostic groups, the quantitative distinction between conductive and sensory components in the individual infant is another matter. At present, there are limited data on the accuracy of such inference with infants.

Yield

In Table 5–2, some recently published results from ABR screening programs are summarized. Several generalities can be gleaned from these data, even though considerable differences, which are not always obvious from such a table, exist between studies. When estimating incidence of a relatively rare disorder, sample size demands are high in order to control the variability of estimates. For example, in a study with 100 cases and an incidence estimate of 0.1 (10 percent), the standard deviation (SD) of the estimate is approximately 0.03 (3 percent). Such an incidence estimate is quite possible, even though the true incidence may be as low as 0.05 or as high as 0.15. For a study with 1000 cases, on the other hand, the SD is under 0.01 (1 percent), other things being equal.

The study by Roberts and associates (1982) is included in Table 5–2 for completeness, although it has been seriously criticized with regard to methodology and low follow-up rate (Fria, 1985; Jacobson and Morehouse, 1984). Disregarding that study, the percentage of screening failure ranges from approximately 10 to 20 percent for screening click intensities of 25 to 40 dB. It is interesting that the failure rates at 40 dB are not generally lower than those at 25 to 30 dB,

Table 5–2.   The Results of ABR Screening and Follow-up in High-Risk Newborns

| | Screen | | | | Retest | |
Study	Failure Cutoff	Number Screened	Number Failed	% Failed	% Retested	% Impaired
Roberts et al. (1982)	40	75	44	58.7	10 (23%)	1.3
Jacobson and Morehouse (1983)	30	176	35	19.9	33 (94%)	4.0
Stein et al. (1983)	40	100	20	20	8 (40%)	2.0
Cevette (1984)	30	745	157	21.1	50 (32%)	7.6
Cox et al. (1984)	30	50	9	18.0	9 (100%)	4.0
Dennis et al. (1984)	30	200	23	11.5	15 (65%)	5.0
Galambos et al. (1984)	30	1613	259	16.1	139 (54%)	4.9
Hyde et al. (1984)	40	303	36	11.9	25 (70%)	4.0
Salamy (1984)	35	2500	414	16.6	176 (43%)	3.2
Shannon et al. (1984)	25	168	21	12.5	19 (90%)	2.2
Finitzo-Hieber et al. (1985)	40	150	33	22.0	27 (81%)	3.3
Fria (1985)	30	500	66	13.2	31 (47%)	4.2
Sanders et al. (1985)	30	1586	266	16.8	N/A	2.7

as noted earlier. This suggests that there may be significant between-study differences in the true failure rates, probably due to technique differences, genuine population differences, or both.

Table 5–2 shows that from 2 to 8 percent of high-risk infants have significant hearing loss on follow-up testing. This is a massive variation in incidence estimates, but there are considerable differences between studies in terms of the types and degrees of hearing loss included in the estimates. As noted previously, there may be large variations in the populations examined. For example, if an ICN includes a large tertiary intake, a high incidence of severe sensory impairment might be expected. Overall, it is noteworthy that the incidences of impairment at follow-up are all above 2 percent, with the exception of that reported by Roberts and associates (1982). The actual figures of severe hearing loss are probably greater than reported in Table 5–2, because these values represent only 60 percent of the initial failures retested. When Schulman-Galambos and Galambos (1975) first reported approximately 1 in 50 high-risk newborns as severely impaired on the basis of ABR measurements, their results were greeted with surprise and skepticism. Subsequent studies have tended to support their results.

Finally, it is clear from Table 5–2 that the rates of successful follow-up vary greatly between studies. Not only is this a potential source of bias in estimates of disease incidence, but it also reveals both the extent and the variability of the compliance problem discussed previously.

Future Directions

Early hearing assessment is likely to become more widely practiced than it is at present, and electrophysiological methods will contribute increasingly to this surge. The ABR is not the only electrophysiological tool available; others include the middle-latency response (MLR), the 40 Hz potential, and electrocochleography. There has already been much research into the comparative accuracy of these and other evoked potential procedures. If the history of other aspects of electric response audiometry is any guide, it seems unlikely that a single evoked potential method will prove to be universally applicable or superior; rather, a strategy incorporating various techniques governed by the features of the individual patient will emerge. The ABR will probably survive as a major component of any such strategy.

The introduction of any major new technique into any area of health care is likely to suffer problems during its "shakedown" phase. Some problems are related to the inevitable evolution of skills and experience with the new technique, uncritical adoption of new "things" as salvation, or defensive rejection of new methods by practitioners of classical methods. No individual or method is invariably correct. The real problem is in putting all the pieces together in the best interests of the patient. Thus, devotees of electrophysiological testing must accept the inevitable limitations of what is merely an electrical correlate of hearing, and devotees of behavioral assessment must accept that their cherished beliefs may be questioned or even overthrown by new techniques.

Finally, we must emphasize that no screening test is the solution per se to the problem of optimal hearing health care in early infancy. A complete *system* is required, and education of parents and relevant professionals about the importance of hearing loss—how to recognize, measure, and treat it—is at least as important as the screening tests themselves.

REFERENCES

Alberti, P. W., Hyde, M. L., Riko K., Corbin, H., and Fitzhardinge, P. M. (1985). Issues in early identification of hearing loss. *Laryngoscope, 95,* No. 4, 373–381.

Cann, J., and Knott, J. (1979). Polarity of acoustic click stimuli for eliciting brainstem auditory evoked responses: A proposed standard. *American Journal of EEG Technology, 19,* 125–132.

Carrel, R. E. (1977). Epidemiology of hearing loss. In S. E. Gerber (Ed.), *Audiology in infancy.* New York: Grune and Stratton.

Cevette, M. S. (1984). Auditory brainstem response testing in the intensive care unit. *Seminars in hearing, 5,* 57–69.

Coats, A. C., and Martin, J. L. (1977). Human auditory nerve action potentials and brainstem evoked responses. *Archives of Otolaryngology, 103,* 605–622.

Cox, L. C. (1985). Infant assessment: Development and age-related considerations. In J. T. Jacobson (Ed.), *The auditory brainstem response.* San Diego: College-Hill Press.

Cox, L. C., Hack, M., and Metz, D. A. (1981a). Brainstem-evoked response audiometry: Normative data from the preterm infant. *Audiology, 20,* 53–64.

Cox, L. C., Hack, M., and Metz, D. A. (1981b). Brainstem evoked response audiometry in the premature infant population. *International Journal of Pediatric Otorhinolaryngology, 3,* 213–224.

Cox, L. C., Hack, M., and Metz, D. A. (1982). Longitudinal ABR in the NICU infant. *International Journal of Pediatric Otorhinolaryngology, 4,* 225–231.

Cox, L. C., Hack, M., and Metz, D. A. (1984). Auditory brainstem response abnormalities in the very low birthweight infant: Incidence and risk factors. *Ear and Hearing, 5,* 47–51.

Dennis, J. M., Sheldon, R., Toubas, P., and McCaffee, M. A. (1984). Identification of hearing loss in the neonatal intensive care unit population. *American Journal of Otology, 5,* 201–205.

Despland, P., and Galambos, R. (1980). The auditory brainstem response (ABR) as a useful diagnostic tool in the intensive care nursery. *Pediatric Research, 14*(2), 154–158.

Downs, D. W. (1982). Auditory brainstem response testing in the neonatal intensive care unit: A cautious response. *American Speech-Language-Hearing Association, 24*(12), 1009–1016.

Doyle, D. J., and Hyde, M. L. (1981). Analogue and digital filtering of auditory brainstem potentials. *Scandinavian Audiology* (Stockholm) *10,* 81–89.

Durieux-Smith, A., Edwards, C. G., Picton, T. W., and MacMurray, B. (1985). Auditory brainstem responses to clicks in neonates. *Journal of Otolaryngology, 14* (Suppl. 14), 12–18.

Durieux-Smith, A., and Jacobson, J. T. (1985). Comparison of auditory brainstem response and behavioral screening in neonates. *Journal of Otolaryngology, 14* (Suppl. 14), 47–53.

Eggermont, J. J. (1983). Physiology of the developing auditory system. In S. Trehub and B. Schneider (Eds.), *Auditory development in infancy.* New York: Plenum Press.

Feinmesser, M., and Tell, L. (1971). Progress report: Evaluation of methods for detecting hearing impairment in infancy and early childhood (U.S.P.H.S.-M.C.H.S. Project 06-48D-2), Department of Otolaryngology, Hadassah Hospital, Jerusalem, Israel.

Feinmesser, M., Tell, L., and Levi, H. (1982). Follow-up of 40,000 infants screened for hearing defect. *Audiology, 21,* 197–203.

Finitzo-Hieber, T. (1982). Auditory brainstem response: Its place in infant audiological evaluations. *Seminars in Speech, Language, and Hearing, 3*(1), 76–87.

Finitzo-Hieber, T., McCracken, G. H., and Clinton-Brown, K. (1985). Prospective controlled evaluation of auditory function in neonates given netilmicin or amikacin. *Journal of Pediatrics, 106,* 129–136.

Fria, T. J. (1985). Identification of congenital hearing loss with the auditory brainstem response. In J. Jacobson (Ed.), *The auditory brainstem response.* San Diego: College-Hill Press.

Fria, T. J., and Doyle, W. J. (1984). Maturation of the auditory brainstem response (ABR): Additional perspectives. *Ear and Hearing, 5*(6), 361–365.

Gafni, M., Sohmer, H., Gross, S., Weizman, Z., and Robinson, M. J. (1980). Analysis of auditory nerve brainstem response (ABR) in very young infants. *Archives of Otorhinolaryngology, 14,* 159–163.

Galambos, R. (1978). Use of the auditory brainstem response (ABR) in infant hearing testing. In S. E. Gerber and G. T. Mencher (Eds.), *Early diagnosis of hearing loss.* New York: Grune and Stratton.

Galambos, R., Hicks, G. E., and Wilson, M. J. (1982). Hearing loss in graduates of a tertiary intensive care nursery. *Ear and Hearing, 3,* 87–90.

Galambos, R., Hicks, G. E., and Wilson, M. J. (1984). The auditory brainstem response reliably predicts hearing loss in graduates of a tertiary intensive care nursery. *Ear and Hearing, 5,* 254–260.

Gerber, S. E., and Mencher, G. T. (1978). *Early diagnosis of hearing loss.* New York: Grune and Stratton.

Gerkin, K. P. (1984). The high risk register for deafness. *ASHA, 26*(3), 17–23.

Hecox, K. (1975). Electrophysiological correlates of human auditory development. In L. B. Cohen and P. Salaplex (Eds.), *Infant perception: From sensation to cognition* (Vol. III). New York: Academic Press.

Hecox, K., and Burkhard, R. (1982). Development dependencies of the human brainstem auditory evoked response. *Annals of New York Academy of Sciences, 388,* 538–556.

Hecox, K., and Cone, B. K. (1981). Prognostic importance of brainstem auditory evoked response after asphyxia. *Neurology, 31,* 1429–1439.

Hecox, K., and Galambos, R. (1974). Brainstem auditory evoked responses in human infants and adults. *Archives of Otolaryngology, 99,* 30–33.

Hecox, K., and Jacobson, J. T. (1984). Auditory evoked potential. In J. Northern (Ed.), *Hearing disorders.* Boston: Little, Brown and Company.

Hyde, M. L. (1985). Frequency-specific BERA in infants. *Journal of Otolaryngology, 14* (Suppl. 14), 19–27.

Hyde, M. L., Riko, K., Corbin, H., Moroso, M., and Alberti, P. W. (1984). A neonatal hearing screening research program using brainstem electric response audiometry. *Journal of Otolaryngology, 13*(1), 49–54.

Jacobson, J. T., and Morehouse, C. R. (1984). A comparison of auditory brainstem response and behavioral screening in high-risk and normal newborn infants. *Ear and Hearing, 5*(4), 247–253.

Jacobson, J. T., Morehouse, C. R., and Johnson, M. J. (1982). Strategies for infant auditory brainstem response assessment. *Ear and Hearing, 3*(5), 263–270.

Jacobson, J. T., Novotny, G. M., and Elliott, S. (1980). Clinical considerations in the interpretation of auditory brainstem response audiometry. *Journal of Otolaryngology, 18,* 462–471.

Jewett, D. L., Romano, M. N., and Williston, J. S. (1970). Human auditory evoked potentials: Possible brainstem components detected on the scalp. *Science, 167,* 1517–1518.

Joint Committee on Infant Hearing, (1982). Position statement. *Pediatrics, 70*(3), 496–497.

Kiang, N., Watanabe, T., Thomas, E., and Clark, L. F. (1965). Discharge patterns of single fibers in the cat's auditory nerve. *Research Monographs* (35). Cambridge, MA: MIT Press.

McClelland, R., and McCrea, R. (1979). Intersubject variability of the auditory evoked brainstem potentials. *Audiology, 18,* 462–471.

McFarland, W. H., and Simmons, F. B. (1980). An automated hearing screening technique for newborns. *Journal of Speech and Hearing Disorders, 45,* 495–503.

Mokotoff, B., Schulman-Galambos, C., and Galambos, R. (1977). Brainstem auditory evoked response in children. *Archives of Otolaryngology, 103,* 38–43.

Northern, J. L., and Downs, M. P. (1984). *Hearing in children* (3rd ed.). Baltimore: Williams and Wilkins.

Parving, A., Elberling, C., and Salomon, G. (1981). ECochG and psychoacoustic tests compared in identification of hearing loss in young children. *Audiology, 20,* 365–381.

Pauwels, H. P., Vogeleer, M., Clements, P. A. R., Rousseeuw, P. J., and Kaufman, L. (1982). Brainstem electric response audiometry in newborns. *International Journal of Pediatric Otorhinolaryngology, 4,* 317–323.

Picton, T. W., Stapells, D. R., and Campbell, K. B. (1981). Auditory evoked potentials from the human cochlea and brainstem. *Journal of Otolaryngology, 10,* (Suppl. 9), 1–41.

Roberts, J. L., Davis, H., Phon, G. L., Reichert, T. J., Sturtevant, E. M., and Marshall, R. E. (1982). Auditory brainstem responses in preterm neonates: Maturation and follow-up. *Journal of Pediatrics, 101,* 257–263.

Salamy, A. (1984). Maturation of the auditory brainstem response from birth through early childhood. *Journal of Clinical Neurophysiology, 1*(3), 293–329.

Salamy, A., Fenn, B. C., and Bronshvag, M. (1979). Ontogenesis of human brainstem evoked potential amplitude. *Developmental Psychobiology, 7,* 519–526.

Salamy, A., and McKean, C. M. (1976). Postnatal development of the human brainstem potentials during the first year of life. *Electroencephalography and Clinical Neurophysiology, 40,* 418–426.

Salamy, A., and McKean, C. M. (1977). Habituation and dishabituation of cortical and brainstem evoked potential amplitude. *International Journal of Neuroscience, 7,* 175–182.

Salamy, A., McKean, C. N., and Buda, F. B. (1975). Maturational changes in auditory transmission as reflected in human brainstem potentials. *Brainstem Research, 96,* 361–366.

Salamy, A., McKean, C. N., Pettett, C., and Mendelson, T. (1978). Auditory brainstem recovery processes from birth to adulthood. *Psychophysiology, 15*(3), 214–220.

Salamy, A., Mendelson, T., Tooley, W. H., and Chaplin, E. R. (1980). Contrasts in brainstem function between normal and high-risk infants in early postnatal life. *Early Human Development, 4*(2), 179–185.

Sanders, R., Durieux-Smith, A., Hyde, M., Jacobson, J., Kileny, P., and Murnane, O. (1985). Incidence of hearing loss in high-risk and intensive care nursery infants. *The Journal of Otolaryngology, 14* (Suppl. 14), 28–33.

Schulman-Galambos, C., and Galambos, R. (1975). Brainstem auditory evoked responses in premature infants. *Journal of Speech and Hearing Research, 18,* 456–465.

Schulman-Galambos, C., and Galambos, R. (1979). Brainstem response audiometry in newborn hearing screening. *Archives of Otolaryngology, 105,* 86–90.

Shannon, D. A., Felix, J. K., Krumholz, A., Goldstein, P. J., and Harris, K. C. (1984). Hearing screening of high-risk newborns with brainstem auditory evoked potentials: A follow-up study. *Pediatrics, 73,* 22–36.

Stapells, D. R., Picton, T. W., Perez-Abalo, M., Reed, D., and Smith, A. (1985). Frequency specificity in evoked potential audiometry. In J. T. Jacobson (Ed.), *The auditory brainstem response.* San Diego: College-Hill Press.

Starr, A., and Achor, L. J. (1975). Auditory brainstem responses in neurological disease. *Archives of Neurology, 32,* 761–768.

Starr, A., Amlie, R. N., Martin, W. H., and Sanders, S. (1977). Development of auditory function in newborn infants revealed by auditory brainstem potentials. *Pediatrics, 60,* 831–839.

Stein, L., Ozdamar, O., Kraus, N., and Paton, J. (1983). Follow-up of infants screened by auditory brainstem response in the neonatal intensive care unit. *Journal of Pediatrics, 103,* 447–453.

Stockard, J. E., and Stockard, J. J. (1981). Brainstem auditory evoked potentials in normal and otoneurologically impaired newborns and infants. In M. Henry (Ed.), *Current clinical neurophysiology* (pp. 421–466). New York: Elsevier—North Holland.

Stockard, J. E., Stockard, J. J., and Coen, R. W. (1983). Auditory brainstem response variability in infants. *Ear and Hearing, 4*(1), 11–23.

Stockard, J. E., Stockard, J. J., Westmoreland, B. F., and Corfits, J. L. (1979). Brainstem auditory evoked response. Normal variations as a function of stimulus and subject characteristics. *Archives of Neurology, 36,* 823–831.

Stockard, J. J., Stockard, J. E., and Sharbrough, F. W. (1978). Nonpathologic factors influencing brainstem auditory evoked potentials. *American Journal of EEG Technology, 18,* 177–209.

Trehub, S. E., Schneider, B. A., and Bull, D. (1981). Effect of reinforcement on infant's performance in an auditory detection task. *Developmental Psychology, 17,* 872–877.

Wilson, W. R., and Thompson, G. (1984). Behavioral audiometry: Children. In J. Jerger (Ed.), *Recent advances in hearing disorders.* San Diego: College-Hill Press.

Chapter 6

Follow-up of Infants in a Neonatal Hearing Screening Program

Laszlo K. Stein

The screening of large numbers of infants for hearing loss may be expected to increase as testing procedures improve and the importance of early detection gains wider acceptance. Implementation of infant hearing screening programs will require not only knowledge of test methodology, the specifics of the test to be used for the detection of hearing loss, but also an understanding of the diagnostic and treatment components essential to the successful screening program.

Follow-up, too often overlooked or treated as an afterthought, is by definition an integral part of the screening process. To quote Thorner and Remein (1982), ''The basic purpose of screening for disease detection is to separate from a large group of apparently well persons those who have a high probability of having the disease under study, *so that they may be given a diagnostic workup and, if diseased, brought to treatment''* (italics added). This widely accepted statement of purpose links the separation of the suspect from the apparently well (the detection process) inextricably with the need for follow-up (the diagnostic and treatment process). Everything done during the separation-detection phase must lead directly to provision of diagnosis and treatment. In fact, without such a direct and planned connection and the promise that health benefits will result from the finding of cases, the advisability of doing a screening test is doubtful, even though it may meet our criteria for simplicity, sensitivity, specificity, and cost-effectiveness. It should always be kept in mind that the ultimate goal of an infant hearing screening program is to help the hearing-impaired child achieve his or her full potential through the timely provision of medical, habilitative, and educational treatment.

In this chapter, the integral nature of follow-up services in screening infants for hearing loss will be emphasized. Focus will be on factors that ensure that the basic purpose of screening, as defined here, is met.

PRELIMINARY CONSIDERATIONS

Basic to any hearing screening program is a considered and thorough determination of whether there truly exists a need for establishing an infant hearing screening program that goes beyond routine use of an at-risk register. As elementary as this may appear, there are a number of compelling reasons why a full-scale infant hearing screening program with its attendant follow-up components may not be warranted or why an alternative might be appropriate.

First, any proposal that originates with the hospital's service auxiliary or community service organization because identifying deaf babies is a worthy eleemosynary project should be viewed with caution. As noble as the intent might be, a decision to launch an infant hearing screening program that involves actual testing and follow-up should proceed only after the professional staff has completed a feasibility study that reviews the experience of comparable facilities and includes a systematic assessment of the hospital's needs and resources.

Probably the most important data that a feasibility study should provide is an estimate of the expected incidence of hearing loss in the newborn population and a projection of the number of infants that would require follow-up services. Because congenital hearing loss is a low-incidence handicap, estimated to be 1 to 2 per 1000 live births, efforts at mass testing and follow-up have tended to focus on the neonatal intensive care unit (NICU), where the incidence of hearing loss has been estimated to be 30 to 50 times greater than in the well-baby nursery (WBN) (Schulman-Galambos and Galambos, 1979; Simmons, 1980). The smaller community hospital with only a WBN and where the number of at-risk births has been the exception may want to consider an alternative to direct testing. One possibility would be initiation of an at-risk register and liaison with a neighboring tertiary care hospital with the capability to test and follow up infants referred as at risk or suspect. This type of regional networking for hearing screening in both rural and urban areas could follow the guidelines that have been established by most states for perinatal special care centers.

By initiating an at-risk register, the hospital with only a WBN can substantially lessen a questionable demand on its resources and still provide a high level of awareness among staff for possible hearing loss in newborns. Support for use of a high-risk register in a WBN is provided by Stein, Clark, and Kraus (1983), who found that approximately half the hearing-impaired infants who received their care in a WBN manifested one of more of the risk factors listed by the Joint Committee on Infant Hearing (1982). If the personnel of the WBN had been aware of the risk criteria, these infants might have been identified as at risk, referred for screening, and, quite possibly, begun therapy at an earlier age.

The availability and vigorous marketing of infant hearing testing instruments, principally auditory brainstem response (ABR) units and automated screening devices that record neonatal motor activity coincident with an auditory signal, have prompted increasing numbers of neonatologists and pediatricians to consider testing in the NICU. Such efforts obviously should be encouraged when such testing is part of a comprehensive hearing screening program that includes follow-up services. Establishing a comprehensive screening service is not, however, without problems. The interdisciplinary nature of the successful infant hearing screening program requires a cooperative effort involving neonatology, audiology, otology, nursing, and quite often the combined staffs of specialty pediatric clinics. In the large tertiary care hospital, such a joint effort may present formidable logistic and administrative challenges. Again, as in the case of the smaller community hospital, a feasibility study is the essential first step. The plan for infant hearing screening in an NICU should consider such population factors as average monthly census, percentage of low birthweight infants, the number of transported or transferred infants, and whether the NICU handles only special problems such as cardiac or surgical cases. Each of these, in combination with the screening level selected, will significantly affect the number of infants who might fail an initial screening and the number who will require follow-up service. The resources of pediatric audiologic and otologic services of the hospital and those of the community for habilitative-educational services, if these are not available within the hospital, should be determined. Additionally, but by no means trivial, are a number of issues relating to program cost, charges, and professional responsibility for over-all direction of the program.

SELECTION OF SCREENING LEVEL

The number of infants requiring diagnostic follow-up testing directly depends on the level at which the screening test is considered positive. Because it is possible to vary the sensitivity and specificity of infant hearing tests by manipulating a variety of test parameters, the consequences of different proportions of false positives and false negatives must be carefully weighed. Selection of a screening level is largely an administrative decision involving value judgments as to the effects of false test results on the screenees and the resources of the program and community.

If the decision is to detect every infant with possible hearing loss regardless of severity, it may be possible to set the screening level low enough to achieve almost 100 percent sensitivity. All infants with a true mild hearing loss will be positive to the test, but many infants in the normal, near-normal, or borderline range will also test as positive, and the test will have poor specificity. The benefits of the high false-positive rate required to identify mild and possibly transitory conditions must be weighed against the possible burden imposed on the diagnostic follow-up services of the program because of the need to test larger numbers of false negatives.

Justification for selection of a screening level involves medical as well as administrative and financial issues. It must be proved that the value of a true positive finding increases the suspect infant's chances of receiving a cure or treatment crucial for his or her future well-being. The detection of hearing loss, in contrast to some other disease conditions, is not dependent upon the setting of a single absolute level that clearly reflects the presence or absence of a potentially handicapping condition. The degree and the nature of a hearing loss, especially in infancy, that constitutes a handicap or potential handicap is still subject to considerable debate. It is not unusual to find medical or educational recommendations for the selection of hearing screening levels that range from the need to detect all infants with hearing loss of 20 dB HL or greater to levels that will detect only those with permanent bilateral sensorineural hearing loss exceeding 60 dB HL. Under such circumstances, compromises on the level of test sensitivity may be sought, and medical or educational issues may often be overshadowed by other factors.

A high false-positive rate may also tend to discredit the screening procedure. Physicians and administrators may question the value of a procedure that falsely alarms parents or that unnecessarily burdens the diagnostic follow-up resources of the facility. The potentially adverse psychological impact on parents of being told that there may be something wrong with the hearing of their infant has not always been carefully considered (Kuyper, 1981; Stein and Jabaley, 1981). A screening level with poor specificity can needlessly alarm large numbers of parents and, fairly or unfairly, discredit the program and jeopardize its continuance. This is especially true if high false test results create lengthy delays between the time of screening and the scheduling of diagnostic testing.

In order to obtain an estimate of the screening level that will yield optimal results for particular hospital or community situations, the number of infants to be screened must be known and sensitivity and specificity data must be available. Direct acquisition of the frequency of false test results is generally beyond the scope of most infant hearing screening programs because of the requirement that a diagnosis of hearing loss be made or ruled out for every infant screened. Knowledge of the false-positive rate associated with commonly used screening levels, however, can be derived from a number of published studies.

Table 6–1 summarizes available published results of ABR screening with NICU infants. Listed are screening levels in dB nHL, initial fail rate in numbers tested (when reported) and percent, the number and percent of infants identified with some degree of hearing loss on follow-up, and the number and percent with severe to profound hearing loss on follow-up. The reader is urged to consult the individual published studies for specific details on SPL reference for screening levels, criteria for fail (audiological and neurological), numbers and percent of screening fails seen for follow-up, and methods used for follow-up testing.

In general, the initial fail rate for 30 or 40 dB nHL click stimulus ranges, with few exceptions, from 15 to 20 percent. The percentage of infants confirmed to have severe to profound sensorineural bilateral loss consistently falls in the 2 to 4 percent range. The number of infants identified as having lesser degrees of hearing loss is not clear, but available figures suggest approximately 5 to 10 percent of the initial fail group may fall in this category.

Miller and Simmons (1984) report a false-positive error rate of 13.83 percent using the Crib-o-gram. This estimate was based on follow-up testing on 36.4 percent of the fail population. A recent study by Durieux-Smith, Picton, Edwards, Goodman, and MacMurray (1985) evaluated the Crib-o-gram test using ABR as the comparison standard. Results of comparison made on 280 infants showed that one third of the infants with normal ABR thresholds failed the Crib-o-gram and that the observed false-negative rate for Crib-o-gram screening decreased when the criterion for passing the ABR was increased to 60 dB nHL.

From published data on both the ABR and automated screening test for neonatal motor activity in response to sound, it is evident that the sensitivity of both can be very high for hearing loss of severe degree. The number of infants requiring diagnostic follow-up services in this instance is appreciably less than when the criterion for fail or screening level is lowered. Balanced against this would be failure to detect potentially handicapping hearing losses of lesser degree. Use of the data shown in Table 6–1 and the published findings with other screening tests on false-positive rates can serve as the basis for clinicians and administrators to approximate the number of infants

Table 6–1. ABR Screening and Follow-Up Results With NICU Infants

Study	Screening Level (dB nHL)	Initial Fail N	Initial Fail %	HL on Retest N	HL on Retest %	Profound HL N	Profound HL %
Despland and Galambos (1980	30	14/91	15.0				
Jacobson et al. (1981)	30	12/83	14.0			3/8	3.6
Cox et al. (1981)	60		12.0				2.3
Galambos et al. (1982)	30	141/890	15.7	43/890	8.9	16/890	1.8
Roberts et al. (1982)	40	44/75	59.0			3/128	2.3
Stein et al. (1983)	40	11/100	11.0				
	60	9/100	9.0	4/99	4.0	2/99	2.0
Galambos et al. (1984)[1]	30	259/1613	16.1		9.1		4.0
Cevette (1984)	30	97/745	13.0		10.4		
	60	60/745	8.0		7.6		2.0
	Abs	30/745	4.6				
Salamy and Amochaev (1984)	20–80[2]	414/2454	16.8	80/2454[3]	3.2		
Sanders et al. (1985)							
Ottawa	30	102/369	27.6	27/369	7.3	7/369	2.0
Halifax	30	43/435	27.5	27/345	7.8	7/345	2.0
Edmonton	25	8/84	9.5			3/84	3.5
Winnipeg	32	73/493	12.9				
Toronto	30		25.0	25/273	9.2	10/273	3.7

[1]Includes data from 1982 study.
[2]Fail level not stated.
[3]Represents a 42.5% follow-up rate (176/414)

that would require diagnostic services in their particular setting. Such a projection, along with careful assessment of the goals and resources available to the program, should be fundamental to any infant hearing screening program.

CONCLUSIONS

This chapter stresses the integral nature of follow-up services in screening infants for hearing loss. Too often, the planning of an infant hearing screening program emphasizes the methodology of detection (the specifics and presumed advantages or disadvantages of using one test over another) with little or no thought given to the provision of diagnosis and treatment. Rather than begin by trying to decide which screening test to use, it might be more appropriate to first give thought to whether the planned program has the resources to meet the promise that health benefits will result from the finding of cases. Without a planned and direct connection between the screening or detection process and the provision of follow-up services, the diagnostic and treatment process, the advisability of performing screening testing is doubtful.

Ensuring that the basic purpose of infant hearing screening is met is dependent upon many factors, ranging from the highly technical to purely administrative and subjective. Several factors were introduced as theoretical issues. In succeeding chapters, these and additional points bearing on implementation of follow-up services are described in practice. These chapters serve as excellent sources, reviewing the experience of facilities that have successfully implemented infant hearing screening programs. Although each describes differing approaches that best meet individual circumstances, all emphasize the interdisciplinary nature of infant hearing screening and the primacy of follow-up services.

REFERENCES

Cevette, M. S. (1984). Auditory brainstem response testing in the intensive care unit. *Seminars in Hearing, 5,* 57–69.

Cox, L. C., Hack, M., and Metz, D. A. (1981). Brainstem evoked response audiometry in the premature infant population. *Journal of Pediatric Otorhinolaryngology, 3,* 213–214.

Despland, P., and Galambos, R. (1980). The auditory brainstem response (ABR) is a useful diagnostic tool in the infant intensive care unit. *Pediatric Research, 14*(2), 1154–158.

Durieux-Smith, A., Picton, T., Edwards, C., Goodman, J. T., and MacMurray, B. (1985). The Crib-o-gram in the NICU: An evaluation based on brainstem electric response and audiometry. *Ear and Hearing, 6,* 20–24.

Galambos, R., Hicks, G. E., and Wilson, M. J. (1982). Hearing loss in graduates of a tertiary intensive care nursery. *Ear and Hearing, 3,* 87–90.

Galambos, R., Hicks, G. E., and Wilson, M. J. (1984). The auditory brainstem response reliably predicts hearing loss in graduates of a tertiary intensive care nursery. *Ear and Hearing, 5,* 254–260.

Jacobson, J. T., Seitz, M. R., Mencher, G. T., and Parrott, V. (1981). Auditory brainstem response: A contribution to infant assessment and management. In G. Mencher and S. Gerber (Eds.), *Early management of hearing loss.* New York: Grune and Stratton.

Joint Committee on Infant Hearing (1982). Position Statement. *Ear and Hearing, 4,* 3–4.

Kuyper, P. (1981). Audiometry and the newborn. *Audiology, 20,* 530–533.

Miller, K., and Simmons, B. (1984). A retrospective and update on the Crib-o-gram neonatal hearing screening audiometer. *Seminars in Hearing, 5,* 49–56.

Roberts, J. L., Davis, H., Phon, G. L., Reichert, T. J., Sturtevant, E. M., and Marshall, R.E. (1982). Auditory brainstem responses in preterm neonates: Maturation and follow-up. *Journal of Pediatrics, 101,* 257–263.

Salamy, A., and Amochaev, A. (1984). A practical approach to hearing screening of the newborn and at-risk infant. *Seminars In Hearing, 5,* 39–47.

Sanders, M. A., Durieux-Smith, A., Hyde, M., Jacobson, J., Kileny, P., and Murnane, O. (1985). Incidence of hearing loss in high-risk and intensive care nursery infants. *Journal of Otolaryngology, 14,* 28–33.

Schulman-Galambos, C., and Galambos, R. (1979). Brainstem response audiometry in newborn hearing screening. *Archives of Otolaryngology, 105,* 86–90.

Simmons, F. B. (1980). Patterns of deafness in newborns. *Laryngoscope, 90,* 448–453.

Stein, L., Clark, S., and Kraus, N. (1983). The hearing-impaired infant: Patterns of identification and habilitation. *Ear and Hearing, 4,* 232–236.

Stein, L., and Jabaley, T. (1981). Early identification and parent counseling. In L. Stein, E. Mindel, and T. Jabaley (Eds.), *Deafness and mental health.* New York: Grune and Stratton.

Stein, L., Ozdamar, O., Kraus, N., and Paton, J. (1983). Follow-up of infants screened by auditory brainstem response in the neonatal intensive care unit. *Journal of Pediatrics, 103,* 447–453.

Thorner, R. M., and Remein, Q. R. (1982). Principles and procedures in the evaluation of screening for disease. In J. B. Chaiklin, I. M. Ventry, and R. F. Dixon (Eds.), *Hearing measurement: A book of readings* (2nd ed.). Reading, MA: Addison-Wesley.

Chapter 7

Considerations in the Implementation of a Hospital-Based Neonatal Hearing Screening Program

Elca T. Swigart

Once a newborn baby leaves the hospital, a considerable period of time elapses before a hearing loss is suspected. Additional time is required for the extent of the hearing loss to be confirmed and habilitation considered. Historically, it has been reported that a child with a severe hearing loss may be over 2 years of age before treatment is begun (Bergstrom, Hemenway, and Downs, 1971). On the other hand, if the possibility of a hearing loss can be detected at birth, the extent of the loss can then be readily identified, and habilitation can be initiated at a much earlier age.

According to the 1980 Vital Statistics (U.S. Department of Health and Human Services, 1980), approximately 99 percent of the births in the United States take place in a hospital setting. Therefore, the hospital nursery, where nearly all babies are available for tests, is a logical place to attempt to identify as many hearing-impaired infants as possible.

There are probably as many variances in hospital administrative structure, support services, and building arrangements as there are hospitals. It follows that the designs of hearing screening programs are likely to be as varied as the hospital settings in which they are established. Therefore, it is not possible to suggest a routine method for establishing a hearing screening program. General factors necessary for screening, as well as those factors that greatly contribute to the success of the entire program, can be identified. These factors should be considered in detail prior to the actual implementation of a neonatal hearing screening program.

INTERPROFESSIONAL AND ADMINISTRATIVE COLLABORATION

Hearing screening is best accomplished by a team approach, with each professional having a vital role in the complete program. Although hospital settings will differ to some degree, each of the following professionals will likely be a participant.

Audiologist

An audiologist must be involved in a neonatal hearing screening program. Although any individual may be instrumental in initiating a screening program, the audiologist is usually best suited to serve as coordinator in light of specialized training and experience in diagnosing and habilitating the hearing impaired.

It is the audiologist who has the experience to interpret screening results and determine appropriate tests to document suspected hearing loss. Furthermore, it is the task of the audiologist to educate each of the other professionals concerning various aspects of the screening program.

Pediatrician

Although historically defined as a ''medical practitioner who specializes in the diseases of children'' (*Stedman's Medical Dictionary,* 1976), the present-day pediatrician also supervises the general development and care of the population he serves. Current medical practice encourages periodic well-baby checks to note growth and development and to identify at the onset any abnormalities or diseases that may impede the optimal developmental process. In light of the complexity of the child and its growth, a pediatrician usually welcomes any noninvasive procedure that can rule out pathology. Not only are the results of a screening test informative, but a high-risk register itself provides useful information. According to Dr. Marcia McCrae, a pediatrician in Reading, Pennsylvania (personal communication, May, 1985), audiological screening in the nursery is an excellent way to detect other disability. Hearing newborns who fail to show normal responses to auditory stimuli may have central nervous system depression or dysfunction. These infants deserve close scrutiny of development and early referral if skills emerge late or with poor quality. The high-risk register may also signal children at jeopardy for mental retardation, cerebral palsy, or learning disability.

Because of the nature of the pediatrician's role as director of the newborn nursery and a general supervisor of the child's development, he must play a major role in the planning of the screening program. Once the program is in operation, he must be informed of all screening results and must also be aware of suggested follow-up evaluations and any diagnostic test results.

Otolaryngologist

The role of the otolaryngologist (also known as otologist or otorhinolaryngologist, based on areas of specialization) is to examine the children who have failed not only the screening but also the follow-up diagnostic testing. The otolaryngologist will consult with the pediatrician concerning those aspects of the child's care that may pertain to the ears. Depending on the interprofessional structure in a pediatric clinic or the working relationship of the pediatrician and otolaryngologist in any given locality, the pediatrician may choose to give medical clearance for amplification or he may refer the child to a specialist. This give-and-take between the pediatrician and otolaryngologist also applies to the treatment of ear disease. In some clinics or community practices, a referral chain may already be established. In other instances, the hearing screening coordinator may assist in establishing a referral system acceptable to all concerned. To avoid unnecessary conflict, the screening coordinator must be aware of the preferences of the professionals and the established referral tracks before designing the screening program.

Neonatologist

Where an intensive care nursery (Level III) is in existence, a neonatologist may be in charge of the over-all nursery; his role is similar to that of the pediatrician. He must be involved in planning the screening program. Because of the multiple involvements of the sick neonates in an intensive care unit, the neonatologist's opinion on when and where to administer screening tests must be considered and respected.

Nursing Supervisor and Staff

Nurses in the newborn nursery become involved in any hearing screening process. Each child's well-being is their responsibility, and any screening process interrupts the nursery routine and invades their working space. However, nurses are usually very willing to cooperate with a screening program if they understand the importance of early detection of hearing loss and if they believe that the coordinator is attempting to interfere as little as possible with their required duties.

Of utmost importance is the nurses' knowledge concerning the test and what the test results really mean. Although the individual administering the test or the screening coordinator may relay the test results to the mother, it is the nurse who the mother will ask later in the day to find out exactly what "that hearing test was all about."

Additional Supportive Personnel

Sometimes other professionals are involved with the screening and follow-up. These people may include trained individuals specializing in child development or the habilitative process. Volunteers are also frequently used to assist in screening. Volunteers must be well informed about the screening process and understand the limitations placed upon them with regard to their volunteer status.

Administrative Staff

It is imperative that the administrative staff understand, approve, and fully support the hearing screening program. Although their formal education may be quite varied, hospital administrators are likely to have received the least amount of information concerning hearing and hearing loss of all professionals associated with the hearing screening program. The coordinator must ensure that the administrators are aware of the importance of early identification of hearing loss and that they understand the goals of screening. They must be apprised of all professional involvements and time requirements. They then can assist in determining costs, locating possible reimbursement sources, and working out the billing routine. Administrative support is invaluable in maintaining interprofessional collaboration.

Basic Concepts to Promote Collaboration

To promote optimum interprofessional collaboration, there are four basic concepts that every professional involved with hearing screening must thoroughly understand.

1. *The importance of early identification.* In almost all areas of pathology, there is an advantage in early diagnosis and treatment. Identification of a hearing loss is no exception. When hearing loss is present in infancy, there is danger that language skills may be delayed or that they may never reach full development. Early identification and treatment can significantly reduce the consequences of a hearing loss. The reader is referred to Chapter 1 of this text for additional information on this topic.

2. *Principles of screening.* It is vital that all professionals understand the principles of screening. The objective of screening is to make a distinction between individuals with a high probability of having a disorder and those who are not likely to have the disorder. Screening is not diagnostic. Those individuals with the high probability of a disorder require additional ''diagnostic'' testing to determine whether or not the disorder actually exists.

   It is intended that hearing screening tests will give negative results when an infant has normal hearing (specificity) and will give positive results when an infant has a hearing loss (sensitivity). At this time, no high-risk register or screening test is 100 percent efficient. Therefore, to fully comprehend the hearing screening process, the professional must realize that in the best screening efforts, there will be some ''false alarms.'' That is, some babies will be identified as having a high probability of a hearing loss who later will be found with normal hearing. There will also be a few babies with a hearing loss who will be ''overlooked'' in the screening process. This means that a few babies will be identified as not having a high probability of hearing loss and will later be found to be hearing impaired. The reader is referred to Chapter 2 of this text for a detailed discussion of screening sensitivity and specificity and ways to reduce false alarms and minimize the number of undetected hearing losses.

3. *Significance of screening results.* With the exception of the administrative staff, all professionals mentioned in this chapter may come in contact with the parent. Therefore, they must know what to tell the parent when the baby does not pass the screening. There is a fine line between alarming the parents and encouraging them to return for follow-up. To avoid any misconceptions, it is important that every professional know exactly what to say. The parents must never be told that their baby has a hearing loss, and the use of the word ''fail'' should be avoided. Instead, parents may be told that the results were not quite as good or as clear as the tester would like them to be. The parents may be given reasons for the child's not responding well. In the case of ABR screening, the child may have been too active, there may have been electrical interference, or there may have been excessive noise in the nursery. In the case of the Crib-o-gram or other behavioral testing, the baby may have recently been fed or may have been in too deep a sleep state to respond well. There may also have been excessive noise in the nursery. Finally, the parents must be informed that it will be necessary to test the child again when he or she is older.

4. *Totality of the screening program.* To be effective, screening is more than the selection of a high-risk register or the purchase of a

piece of equipment and the administration of many tests. There must also be plans to report results, carry out further testing, and finally habilitate those infants found with hearing losses. All professionals must be aware of what is planned and how the plans are to be carried out. They should also be aware of alternate screening procedures and understand why a specific one was selected. In order to achieve full support for the hearing screening, every professional should not only understand every aspect of the proposed program but should also have a voice in its design.

SELECTION OF A SCREENING METHOD

The reader is referred to Chapter 2 of this text for a detailed discussion of selecting a screening method. The main considerations will be briefly mentioned here. First, the population to be screened must be identified. Will it be a well-baby nursery or an intensive care nursery? The target population may be a prime consideration in the selection of test equipment. A reliable, cost-effective method of screening for neonates in an intensive care nursery may not be efficient for screening in a large, well-baby nursery and vice versa. Each of several methods of screening demonstrates merit in given situations. The methods discussed in this text are limited to those most widely used in the United States at the present time. Other test instruments are available, and the reader is encouraged to consider any screening tool in view of the guidelines discussed in Chapter 2.

A second consideration in test selection is the degree of hearing loss to be identified. Resources must be available to carry out follow-up of all referrals from the screening. If mild transient losses are to be identified, there will be many referrals, and some of the infants will be found with normal hearing at a later date. If only moderate or more severe losses are to be identified, there will be fewer referrals, but the milder transient or permanent losses will most likely go undetected. To maintain the credibility of the screening program, those involved must understand precisely what is being identified through the screening process.

Third, personnel to supervise and carry out the actual screening must be available. Are they already at hand or must they be acquired? When limited personnel appear to be a prohibitive factor in implementing a screening program, volunteers can sometimes be successfully used. The use of volunteers has its advantages and limitations. Most volunteers are highly motivated and dedicated individuals; however, they must be recruited, trained, and supervised. In addition, non-staff members have restrictions in a hospital setting.

Fourth, financial support for equipment and the execution of the program must eventually be located. In selecting the test method, the coordinator should be conscious of cost and be alert for possible revenue sources. However, appropriate selection of a screening method and a well-planned program precede the acquisition of financial maintenance.

DETAILS OF THE SCREENING PROCESS

Attention to the details involved with the screening process is a prerequisite of an effective program. Factors that must be considered are included in the check list in Table 7–1 and are discussed below.

Information for Parents

A hearing screening program can serve a vital role in professional and lay education concerning the importance of early identification of hearing loss. It is wise to inform parents about the role hearing plays in the acquisition of speech and language and the importance of detecting hearing loss as early as possible. The screening program and the meaning of the test results should also be made clear. Many centers also find it helpful to inform parents how a normally developing baby should react to sound at different age levels. All this information can be conveniently conveyed by a form letter or pamphlet. The design of either should be attractive, and the information should be concisely but clearly stated in simple language. Remember that individuals of all educational levels have babies.

High-Risk Register

What items will be on the high-risk register? It may be wise to initially select a basic established register such as that recommended by the 1982 Joint Committee on Infant Hearing and described in Chapter 3. If there are particular items that a hospital or physician may wish to investigate, any number of possible high-risk items may be added with the mutual consent of all concerned.

Who will fill out the register? There are two fundamental portions of a register, and information must be obtained from two different sources: (1) The mother must be interviewed to determine family history of hearing loss and the possibility of perinatal infection. Although hereditary factors are complex and require in-depth investi-

TABLE 7–1. Check List for Organizing the Screening Procedure

Parent information (pamphlet or letter)
  Who will distribute ____

High-risk register
  What items are included ____
  Who will obtain information _______________________________________
    Interview mother ____
    Check baby's chart ____
    Obtain release of information (for volunteers)
  Who will record results in hospital chart _________________________
  Who will report results to coordinator ____________________________
    How . . . . Phone _______________ Written message _______________

Screening Test
  Parental consent required . . . . Yes ☐ No ☐
    If yes, who will obtain it ____
  Who will administer the test ______________________________________
  When will testing be done ____
  Where will testing be done ____
    Must baby be transported . . . . Yes ☐ No ☐
      If yes, who will do it ____
  Where will equipment be stored ____________________________________
    Sterilized . . . . How _______________ By whom _______________
  If ABR used,
    Are norms established . . . . Yes ☐ No ☐

Test Results
  Who will interpret ____
  Who will record results in hospital chart _________________________
  How will results be given to coordinator __________________________
  Who will tell parents ____

Reports
  Where to send
    Pediatrician . . . . Yes ☐ No ☐
    Clinic . . . . Yes ☐ No ☐
    Other . . . . Yes ☐ No ☐

Billing
  Who will initiate billing ____
  How ____

gation to determine their true nature, many centers regard genetic traits related to hearing loss in siblings, parents, grandparents, aunts, uncles, and first cousins as positive family history. (2) The baby's chart must be checked to identify items that may suggest a risk for hearing loss. This information may be obtained by any hospital staff member. Some programs use volunteers to assist in this aspect of screening. To protect the confidentiality of the patients, most hospitals permit only staff members to have access to the records. Therefore, if volunteers are used for completing the register, a release of information from the mother is sometimes required. The coordinator should check with the hospital administration for the necessity of a release and the use of the appropriate form.

How will the results of the high-risk register be recorded in the baby's chart and reported to the individual who will do the screening test? This can most readily be accomplished by the individual checking the chart for risk factors. Results can be a hand written note in the appropriate section of the chart or a total sheet containing the high-risk check list added to the chart. Referral for further testing for those at risk may be made by written message or phone contact.

Screening Test

In many hospitals, parental consent must be obtained prior to any hearing screening test. The coordinator should check with the hospital administration on this policy and then, if necessary, determine who will obtain it.

Who will administer the actual screening test? The audiologist is a likely choice in many programs. In some situations, nurses can administer the test; however, this is usually not possible due to the complexity of the test itself or the time limitations of the nurses' schedules. If volunteers or nurses are used, they must be trained and supervised.

When will the testing be done? Testing time must be arranged with the coordinator, the physician, and the nursing supervisor and staff. In most hospitals, nurseries are very active in the early morning hours with rounds and other nursery activities. During these active times, attempts to screen would interfere with the ongoing nursery routine, and the noise levels would prohibit reliable test results. Therefore, late forenoon or afternoon may be a more appropriate time for hearing screening. If ABR is the test selected for screening, it may be wise to check the feeding schedules and screen shortly after feeding when the baby usually falls asleep. With behavioral screening, it is best to avoid the times right after feeding when the baby is generally less responsive.

Where will the testing be done? A quiet area of the nursery will usually suffice, because most equipment for screening is portable. If ABR is the instrument of choice, there may be situations in which the baby must be transported to the space where permanent equipment is located. In this case, it must be predetermined as to who is responsible for transferring the baby and when.

Where will the equipment be stored? Test equipment should be readily accessible yet not interfere with routine nursing activity. Although equipment is usually stored in clean condition, it must be determined when and how the equipment itself or any attachments will be sterilized prior to use with neonates.

At this time, no adequate standards for neonatal ABR data are available. This means that it is not yet possible to compare data between centers. If ABR is the chosen screening instrument, the coordinator must ensure that a control sample of data is obtained on presumably healthy, full-term infants.

Results

Results of some screening tests such as Crib-o-gram require little interpretation to determine whether or not the infant passed the test. Other test results such as that of ABR testing are more involved and do require some form of interpretation. The interpretation should be made by an audiologist or other individual who has had extensive training in the administration of the test as well as in the interpretation of test results.

Who is responsible for recording the results of the screening in the baby's hospital chart? If no interpretation is necessary, the person administering the test may record the results and notify the coordinator by phone or written message. If the results require interpretation, obviously they cannot be recorded until that interpretation has been made. In this case, either the interpreter or someone he designates can make the chart notation and notify the coordinator.

Who will tell the parents? Any individual involved in the screening program can be designated to tell the parents the test results. However, if the child does not pass the test, careful consideration must be made with respect to the message actually conveyed to the parents.

Reports

What will be reported? The results of the screening obviously need to be made known. In addition any intended follow-up should be indicated in terms of when, where, and for what reason.

Where should reports be sent? The child's pediatrician must be apprised of all testing and test results. If the child is being followed by a specialized clinic or a well-baby clinic, results of the screening should also be sent there.

Who will send the reports? The appropriate clerical staff must be designated in advance of starting the screening program.

Billing

Determining the cost of the screening program is discussed in detail in Chapter 10. In addition, there is the matter of billing for the test administered. Usually, the person who charts the results also initiates the billing. This must be discussed with the appropriate administrative staff in the hospital's accounting office.

FOLLOW-UP

A hearing screening program can only be as effective as the follow-up testing and early habilitation of the child identified with a hearing loss. Therefore, there is little value in screening if follow-schedules have not been explicitly identified prior to the initiation of the program.

The screening coordinator may wish to check whether or not the child will be returning to the hospital clinic for medical follow-up. If so, the audiological follow-up may be accomplished at the same time. Discussion with the medical clinic coordinator will assist in determining the manner in which the child will be tagged for audiological testing and sent to the appropriate areas for these tests as part of each medical clinic visit.

If the child will receive medical checks at a physician's office away from the hospital setting, it may be necessary to schedule return visits specifically for audiological evaluation. This possibility should be discussed with the child's pediatrician, so that he or she can be made aware of all scheduled audiological follow-up appointments. A supportive pediatrician can be instrumental in encouraging the parents to return for follow-up audiological tests.

More than one audiological evaluation may be necessary to confirm a hearing loss. Therefore, a routine should be established for both passes and failures at each audiological check. This may include periodic rechecks, medical referral, or referral for habilitative procedures.

When the extent of the hearing loss is confirmed and it is believed that amplification may be of value, medical clearance for the use of amplification must be obtained. In the previous section of this chapter, the procedures for obtaining this medical clearance are discussed.

Once amplification has been provided, the child should be placed in a habilitative program for hearing-impaired infants. These early intervention programs are usually parent and home centered and attempt to assist the parent in providing rich stimulation during the critical speech and language development years. Frequently, placement in the program coincides with the amplification fitting process. Information from parents and people who work with the child is of great value in determining the appropriate hearing aid fitting.

RECORD KEEPING

The screening coordinator must keep records and review them periodically to determine the efficacy of the screening process. It is generally expected that the number of births, the number at risk, the number screened, and the number passing and failing the screening will be recorded. The coordinator must also identify the number of babies actually found with a hearing loss in the follow-up process.

In addition, the coordinator may wish to identify the high-risk factors for those requiring follow-up as well as for those actually identified with hearing loss. There are numerous other possibilities for obtaining relevant information if data are routinely recorded and periodically analyzed. These kinds of records are indispensable in making appropriate adjustments in the screening protocol as the need arises. The information is also useful in justifying these changes to others involved with the program.

COST AND REIMBURSEMENT

Factors to consider in estimating the cost of a screening program are discussed in detail in Chapter 10. Briefly, they include the cost of the equipment, personnel time, supplies, and the hospital overhead or operating expenses.

Reimbursements for actual charges billed usually come from three main sources: (1) private payment, (2) insurance coverage, and (3) state agencies. The total cost of the program may also be reduced by contributions from service organizations or businesses in the local area. Not infrequently, equipment for testing is donated to the program. The coordinator may investigate all sources of financial revenue. However, it should be kept in mind that those funds derived from donations may be temporary or inconsistent unless a great deal of time and effort is spent in promoting public relations to acquire them.

SUGGESTIONS FOR IMPLEMENTING THE PROGRAM

As suggested in the beginning of this chapter, no two hearing screening programs will be alike. Therefore, the implementation of the programs will differ in various aspects. Nevertheless, there are some general approaches that may apply in almost any setting.

It is vital that the program is well planned in advance. Everyone concerned must know what is going to happen, how it is going to happen, and why it is going to happen before the program is put into operation.

At the onset, it is usually wise to let the hospital administration know that you are interested in establishing a hearing screening program. Tell the administration that in order to determine the feasibility of such a program with as little interruption of established hospital routine as possible, you would like to do some investigating. After preliminary permission is granted, ask the administration for the order in which those likely to be involved in the program should be contacted.

Generally, observation and initial planning will start at the nursery level and expand in the general direction of supervisory authority. As an example, it would be very difficult to convince the nursery supervisor that hearing screening can fit into the nursery routine if you have no idea what that routine really is. However, it is strongly advised that you never enter an area without the supervisor's permission and knowledge of your purpose.

The following suggestions will illustrate one possible approach in the development of a screening program and is for illustrative purposes only. It is to be expected that this order may be altered to meet the needs of the hospital and the individual coordinating the program.

It is first necessary to determine how many births occur each year in the target population that you intend to screen. From information reported in the literature, estimate how many infants will be at risk based on the birth census. This may range from a small number for a well-baby nursery to a much larger number for a Level III (sick-baby) intensive care nursery. Have in mind a basic high-risk register and an idea of the test method you would like to use. With the nursing supervisor's permission, go into the nursery and observe its standard routine. Determine the quietest times of day and ask the nurses how you could screen with as little interference in their routine as possible. Locate the medical information to fill out the high-risk register and estimate the time needed to acquire that information for each child.

Talk with the pediatrician and neonatologist. Tell them of the importance of early identification of hearing loss and indicate how a hearing screening program may be possible with minimal interference in the nursery. Ask their opinions on ways to report screening results and arrange follow-up testing. This may also be a time to talk with other involved personnel such as the otologist or specialist in the intensive care nursery.

At this time, it may be appropriate to try out the actual screening tool that you intend to use. Frequently, equipment can be borrowed or placed on trial from a manufacturer. But keep in mind that you never attempt any procedure without the consent of the nursing supervisor and the approval of the child's pediatrician, neonatologist, and hospital administration. Before any testing is administered with electrical equipment, it is imperative that a safety check of the equipment be made by the hospital biomedical staff.

Make as detailed a plan as possible. Check the practicality of what you have proposed with the nursing supervisor, the nursing staff, the pediatrician, the neonatologist, and other involved professionals. Solicit opinions and suggestions and make changes when advisable.

At this time, you are able to estimate the cost of the screening procedure by noting the cost of the equipment and the personnel and time involved to test the estimated number expected to be at risk. Some additional costs, such as that for printing pamphlets may also be included. You should also have looked into possible reimbursement sources or contributions.

Determine possibilities for audiological follow-up and habilitation. Learn how most infants will be followed medically and, if possible, attempt to arrange audiological follow-up to coincide. Locate established habilitative services for the hearing impaired in the community and determine whether special effort is necessary to devise an early intervention program responsive to the needs of the very young infant.

Make the final draft of the hearing screening program as detailed as possible for presentation to the hospital administration. Ask for their opinions and suggestions, and make changes if necessary.

With final administrative approval and the establishment of normative data when appropriate, the screening program can begin. As the program gets under way, listen for opinions, ask for suggestions, and make changes when necessary.

SUMMARY

Hospital-based neonatal hearing screening is a complex endeavor that requires interprofessional and administrative cooperation. ''Planning'' may be considered the most important factor in the establishment of the program. It is time consuming and quite frequently challenging. However, the rewards more than compensate for the time and effort spent in the planning stages.

Because of the multifaceted aspect of hearing screening, the best laid plans may need to be modified as circumstances arise. These modifications should be viewed as stages in an ongoing effort to more efficiently identify and habilitate the hearing-impaired infant. Most importantly, it is hoped that all programs will be designed to allow improvements as new and better screening techniques become known.

REFERENCES

Bergstrom, L., Hemenway, W. G., and Downs, M. P. (1971). A high-risk registry to find congenital deafness. *Otolaryngologic Clinics of North America, 4,* 369–399.

Stedman's medical dictionary (23rd ed.) (1976). Baltimore: Williams and Wilkins.

U.S. Department of Health and Human Services. (1980). *Vital statistics of the United States: Volume I—natality* (DHHS Publication No. PHS 85-1100). Washington, DC: U.S. Government Printing Office.

Chapter 8

Large-Scale High-Risk Neonatal Hearing Screening

Thomas M. Mahoney

It is generally recognized that newborn high-risk hearing screening is an extremely worthwhile public health endeavor. Risk registers reportedly increase the identification sensitivity of mass screening by as much as 35 times (Northern and Downs, 1974) and have the capacity to identify up to 80 percent of all severe to profound hearing impaired newborns (Altman, 1968; Bergstrom, Hemenway, and Downs, 1971; Feinmesser, Tell, and Levi, 1982; Salmivalli, Suonpaa, Johansson, and Jauhiainen, 1980). If such registers were universally implemented, the majority of hearing-impaired neonates could be diagnosed shortly after birth, thereby gaining the advantage of early intervention during the critical language acquisition period from birth to 2½ years of age (Lenneberg, 1967). Importantly, when compared with later intervention, early intervention with hearing-impaired infants has been shown to significantly improve communicative skills (Clark, 1980), which are basic to future psychosocial, educational, and vocational development. In this light, the pressing challenge facing health care professionals is to develop early identification programs that warrant application to large general newborn populations.

In 1972, the Joint Committee on Infant Hearing recommended universal implementation of newborn high-risk screening, and, since that time, a variety of screening methods have been reported (Ehrlich, Shapiro, Kimball, and Henther, 1973; Feinmesser and Tell, 1976; Feinmesser et al., 1982; Fitch, Williams, and Etienne, 1982;

This material originally appeared in *Seminars in Hearing,* 5(1), 25–36. New York: Thieme-Stratton, Inc., 1984. It has been updated for this publication.

Gerber, 1976; Hirsch and Kankkunen, 1974; Mencher, 1974, 1975; Meyer and Wolfe, 1975; Salmivalli et al., 1980; Stewart, 1974). Unfortunately, most of these are private projects that affect a relatively small number of newborns in selected hospitals and, as yet, do not have a significant impact on the total number of unidentified hearing-impaired newborns in the general population.

In addition to a growing number of hospital-based risk registers for well-baby nursery populations, there is an increasing concern about the hearing of newborn intensive care patients. Even though controversy surrounds the preferable identification technique or follow-up protocol (Downs, 1982; Galambos, Hicks, and Wilson, 1982; Marshall, Reichert, Kerley, and Davis, 1980; Simmons, 1982), the very high-risk condition of tertiary intensive care infants spawns a general agreement that their hearing should in some manner be monitored. Because intensive care is necessitated for only approximately 6 percent of the total newborn population (Budetti, Barrand, McManus, and Heiner, 1981) and individual hospital risk registers now in use also cover only a small percentage of the total newborn population in a given geographic area, the majority of neonates in North America remain unscreened.

Since the most frequently occurring risk factor for profound deafness in a general population is positive family history of hearing loss (Mahoney, 1984), the majority of deaf newborns are otherwise healthy, normal-looking babies. Consequently, they pass traditional physical examinations and are often not diagnosed as hearing impaired until 2½ to 3 years of age, or about two years after intervention should ideally begin. With this in mind, it seems that debate centered on test protocols for obvious target populations, such as newborn intensive care survivors, misses a major problem facing early identification today: how to most efficiently, effectively, and economically screen all newborns for hearing impairment at an age early enough to implement optimal habilitation.

The need to screen the hearing of all newborns by a high-risk register was recognized in 1974 at a meeting of international authorities on early identification. As published in 1975 by Mencher, the Nova Scotia Conference resolved: "A high-risk register or file should be universally implemented on the basis of the five points of the Joint Committee on Infant Hearing and the follow-up procedures of that statement should also be universally implemented. We recommend that the World Health Organization, national and local governments adopt this program by legal mandate."

There are at present seven high-risk factors identified by the Joint Committee's 1982 statement. These are the following:

1. A family history of childhood hearing impairment.

2. Congenital perinatal infection (e.g., cytomegalovirus, rubella, herpes, toxoplasmosis, syphilis).
3. Anatomical malformations involving the head or neck (e.g., dysmorphic appearance, including syndromal and nonsyndromal abnormalities, overt or submucous cleft palate, morphological abnormalities of the pinna).
4. Birthweight less than 1500 gm.
5. Hyperbilirubinemia at level exceeding indications for exchange transfusion.
6. Bacterial meningitis, especially from *Haemophilus influenzae* infection.
7. Severe asphyxia, which may include infants with Apgar scores of 0 to 3 who fail to institute spontaneous respiration by 10 minutes and those with hypotonia persisting to 2 hours of age.

The involvement of governmental agencies in mass newborn high-risk hearing screening has monumental implications for early identification. Public health efforts can offer the coordination necessary to effect screening and follow-up of all newborns in large geographic areas. In 1975, it was estimated that only 1 percent of the live births in the United States were screened by a hearing risk register (Mencher, 1975), whereas, by 1981, the coverage increased to approximately 6.8 percent of the total newborn population (Beck, 1981). The 1981 data were based on programs known to be operational by various state governmental agencies. Since the Beck study, additional states have implemented large-scale high-risk screening, and other states have begun either regional projects or are planning statewide efforts. Fortunately, the trend toward early identification and intervention for the hearing impaired seems to be gaining momentum. Even in times of severe competition for health care monies, governmental agencies are beginning to recognize that early identification of hearing loss is clearly in the domain of public health care. This initiative will be directly responsible for the early identification of a growing number of hearing-impaired infants in the general newborn population.

A SURVEY OF GOVERNMENTAL HIGH-RISK HEARING SCREENING PROGRAMS

The author was asked to arrange a session on high-risk hearing screening at the National Meeting of Directors of Speech and Hearing Programs in State Health and Welfare Agencies (DSHPSHWA), held in Toronto, Ontario, on November 16 and 17, 1982. The major purpose of this session was to have representatives of various states and provinces present their high-risk hearing screening programs to the general audience, which was composed of many directors of government speech and hearing agencies. It was hoped that this information sharing would assist those agencies interested in beginning high-risk screening and would generate such an interest for those who had no immediate screening plans.

To implement this goal, a letter inviting participation in the high-risk session was sent to all state and provincial health and welfare departments. Responses indicating a desire to present data on their high-risk programs were subsequently received from representatives of Massachusetts, Georgia, New Jersey, Oklahoma, Arkansas, Alaska, Alabama, Colorado, Nova Scotia, and British Columbia. The author reported on the Utah program. The individual presenters were requested to write short summaries of their programs to help establish a geographical profile of high-risk hearing screening in governmental agencies.

In the summer of 1983, a conference was held in Birmingham, Alabama, to concentrate on several areas of need in speech and hearing in children. One topic was high-risk hearing screening. Sponsored by the United States Department of Health and Human Services, the purpose of the conference was to discuss state of the art knowledge in several target areas and to generate recommendations that would help to establish guidelines for service providers. In preparation for the Alabama conference, the author became aware of several additional efforts to initiate programs in states not represented in Toronto. California, Ohio, Maryland, and Connecticut were reported to have programs in various planning stages; Florida had begun a 2-year regional pilot study; and Tennessee began a regional registry based on birth certificate data. More recently, it was learned that Wisconsin and Arizona have also begun planning government coordinated newborn hearing screening programs and that the Tennessee regional program has expanded statewide.

Figure 8–1 geographically indicates those states and provinces known to have government coordinated statewide or regional high-risk screening programs either in operation or planned as of January 1985. Because the figure represents a composite summary of data obtained from numerous sources, some inconsistencies may exist by the time of printing. The map excludes many excellent hospital-based screening efforts throughout the country under private administration. To assist individuals wishing to obtain information from specific states outlined in Figure 8–1, a list of pertinent addresses is included in Appendix 8–A.

Connecticut, Texas, New Jersey, Massachusetts, Oklahoma, Georgia, California, and Florida have a legislated mandate. Such laws, however, do not always guarantee proper program implementation. As is evident in several states, legal mandates are not necessar-

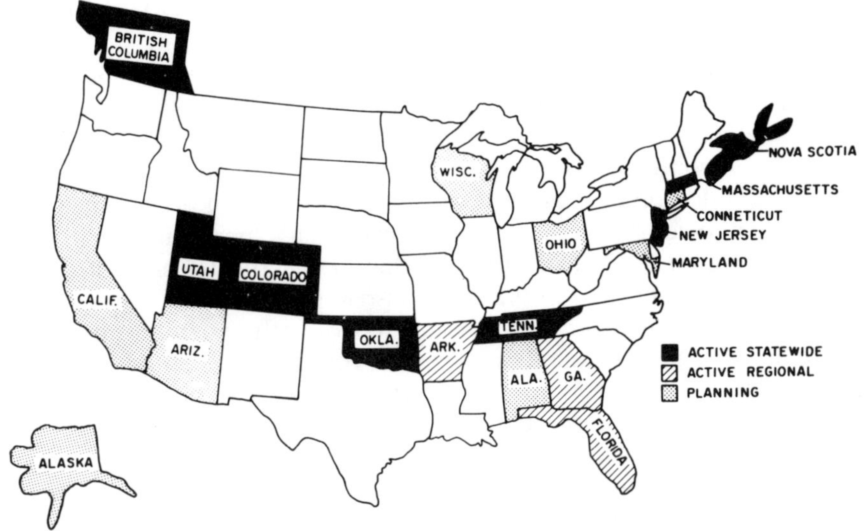

Figure 8–1. States and provinces known to have operative or planned statewide or regional high-risk hearing screening programs.

ily accompanied by financial backing, and, consequently, mandated programs may stagnate for years without funding. In politically conservative states, the attempt but failure to produce legislation may in fact hinder existing or subsequent government or private sector screening.

States and provinces with active regional or statewide programs can be dichotomized into those using the birth certificate for high-risk data and those obtaining initial registry information by some variation of a hospital questionnaire. The following will highlight some of the more developed programs in each of these categories, detailing those that have specific high-risk data or unique programmatic characteristics or both. It is hoped that this information will be of assistance to those readers in a position to initiate new and innovative screening efforts.

PROGRAMS USING BIRTH CERTIFICATE DATA

Utah

In 1978, the Utah Department of Health began using the official birth record as the basis for identifying newborns at risk for hearing loss. In that year, the following question was printed on the birth certificate: ''Has a close relative of the baby had a hearing loss that has existed since childhood?'' That question, together with low Apgar scores and birthweight below 1500 gm, served as the program's three high-risk factors. Beginning with 1983 births, congenital anomalies of the head and neck, hyperbilirubinemia, congenital perinatal infections, and bacterial meningitis were included as risk factors, as recommended by the 1982 Joint Committee on Infant Hearing. Addition of these risk factors to the program necessitated a nosologist to computer code the birth certificates' health information section. Figure 13–2 in Chapter 13 highlights the birth certificate questions pertinent to the current high-risk program.

After excluding infant deaths up to 4 months postpartum, the parents of high-risk infants are sent a computer-generated packet containing an explanation of the program, an educational leaflet about normal infant auditory development, and a postage-paid return card on which a hearing screening appointment may be requested. Nonrespondents receive a second notice in 2 months. Hearing screening is scheduled at one of four state audiology centers or eight traveling clinic sites at no charge to the parents. At the centers, testing involves a one-half hour appointment using a visual reinforcement conditioned response procedure. Auditory brainstem response testing is performed when indicated. Once hearing loss is confirmed, medical clearance for amplification is obtained, hearing aids are prescribed on a trial basis, and weekly home intervention is begun through the Utah Parent-Infant Program (PIP). A statewide service, this program trains parents in methods of language habilitation for their hearing-impaired infant. There is no legislative mandate for the program; it operates under a statute allowing the use of birth certificate data for health and statistical purposes. The 1984 program costs, exclusive of audiological testing, are estimated to be approximately $1.25 per live birth, or $51,000 per year. Maternal and Child Health (MCH) block grant funds are used through the Bureau of Communicative Disorders. From 1978 to 1983, more than 205,000 Utah live births were screened with more than 22,000 (9 percent) infants identified as at risk. After a 50 percent cumulative mailer response, more than 3,000 of these infants were tested at state facilities. Nearly 900 were found to have middle ear involvement, and 77 were diagnosed as having severe or profound bilateral sensorineural hearing loss. Positive family history was the most frequently occurring single high-risk factor in the sensorineural hearing loss group, followed by low birthweight and low Apgar scores. A more detailed description of these data and the total Utah program is presented in Chapter 13.

Georgia

Since 1981, Georgia has had a 16-county regional high-risk hearing screening pilot program based on a combination of birth certificate information and a voluntary hospital referral form. Newborns with positive family history, anoxia, low birthweight, congenital malformations of the head and neck, certain perinatal infections, ototoxic therapy, elevated bilirubin levels, or meningitis are screened. Affected infants can receive behavioral audiometric examinations at local health departments. According to Loyd and Hankla (1983), 384 (4.6 percent) of 8,400 live births in 1982 and 1983 were at risk. Of these, 56 percent were followed for positive family history, 18 percent for low Apgar scores, and 11 percent for low birthweight. Of these infants, 236 had their hearing examined at their local health departments, and 7 were diagnosed as having significant bilateral hearing loss by 1 year of age. Two of the hearing-impaired infants had congenital malformations, one had ototoxic therapy history and congenital malformation, one had low birthweight and congenital malformation, one had positive family history, one had a low Apgar score, and one was identified at risk by elevated bilirubin. This excellent regional program in Georgia has proved to be effective and is expected to be expanded statewide in the near future.

Tennessee

Tennessee has instituted statewide high-risk hearing screening using birth certificate information. Financed through the Department of Health and Environment, Speech and Hearing Services, this effort relies heavily on local department cooperation with the regional Speech and Hearing program. Birth certificates are reviewed for the risk factors recommended by the 1982 Joint Committee on Infant Hearing. Letters recommending hearing screening, along with educational material, are sent to parents of all at-risk infants. A follow-up letter is mailed 6 months after birth to nonrespondents. Behavioral hearing screening is scheduled immediately after response to either letter. Hearing screening is active statewide in all 10 regional health offices. It is planned that by July 1985, a comprehensive high-risk registry for handicapping conditions, incorporating the hearing high-risk register, will be initiated. This computerized registry will allow for efficient case management of all children identified at risk, including infants at risk for hearing impairment. There are no specific data available at this time.

PROGRAMS USING A HOSPITAL QUESTIONNAIRE

Although hospital maternal high-risk questionnaires have been reported to present problems (Mahoney and Eichwald, 1979), many states use some variation of them to implement a hearing risk registry. The birth certificate format is often difficult to change, and, under certain state statutes, birth certificate use is illegal for personal health follow-up. Also, one may sometimes question the accuracy of certain information recorded on birth certificates (Green, Nelson, Gaylor, and Holson, 1979), especially on those items requiring written medical information. It is generally accepted, however, that screening a state's total live births in one central location by computer search of birth records is decidedly more efficient than enlisting and maintaining cooperation from many individual hospitals.

British Columbia

In spite of the extra effort necessitated, some excellent high-risk hearing screening programs rely on hospital newborn maternal questionnaires. Probably one of the most refined is that operated through the Provincial health resources of British Columbia, Canada, by the Division of Speech and Hearing, Ministry of Health. As reported by FitzZaland (1985), the program began in 1975 and has grown so that 20 audiology clinics and 28 hospitals throughout the Province now participate. It is administered through regional public health centers because of the large area of the Province and the scattered population. A high-risk hearing register card is completed in the hospital for all live births and forwarded to the regional audiology center for review and appropriate action. The family physician is advised of any infant determined to be at risk and an audiological evaluation is scheduled at approximately 5 to 7 months of age. Once hearing impairment is confirmed, hearing aids are prescribed. Any infant at risk due to nonbacterial intrauterine fetal infection or hereditary or syndrome factors that could result in progressive hearing impairment is followed by the audiologist. The program is administered as part of total care that includes diagnostic assessment, hearing aid evaluation, fitting and dispensing, speech pathology, and other public health services. Family counseling, individualized education plans, and public information programs are all extensions of the infant identification program. Of 52,858 infants screened in 8 years, 2,695 (5.1 percent) were determined to be at risk, of which 571 (21.2 percent) were identified as hearing impaired. Of the hearing impaired, 80 percent were found to have a conductive hearing loss (48 percent mild, 32 percent moderate), and 13 percent had a sensorineural loss (3 percent mild, 4 percent moderate, 5 percent severe, 1 percent profound). The remaining 7 percent were diagnosed with a mixed hearing impairment (3 percent mild, 2 percent moderate, 1.5 percent severe, 0.5 percent profound). High-risk item analysis shows 59.1 percent of the hearing impaired were at risk by family history, 9.8 percent by rubella or other nonbacterial intrauterine fetal infection, 12 percent by first arch syndrome, 3.1 percent by high bilirubin level, 16 percent by low birthweight. Cost per infant screened, including all administrative and personnel expenses, was $4.93 in 1982 Canadian currency, with a $456.00 overall average expenditure per infant identified.

Massachusetts

Massachusetts has perhaps the oldest state statute requiring newborn hearing screening. Since 1971, state law requires that parents of every child born in a hospital within the state receive information ''describing those conditions which cause certain children to be placed in a high-risk category for hearing impairment.'' They receive a brochure that lists eight high-risk criteria and indicates where to call for further information. The law provides for the evaluation of any high-risk child at state expense at a state-approved evaluation center. Hospital maternity units are required to collect data for all infants and return it to the Department of Public Health. Parents of infants with positive risk factors are contacted by the Department and arrangements are made for audiological evaluations. Services are available to the family until a diagnosis is made or until the child's third birthday. Complete audiological reports are obtained from the evaluation centers and appropriate recommendations for amplification and habilitation are made as needed. The program provides extensive in-service training aimed at improving awareness of the risk factors among nurses, physicians, and social service staff members. Figures from fiscal year 1983 indicate approximately 700 initial evaluations conducted on infants referred through the program. Specific incidence and risk-related data are unavailable at this time.

New Jersey

New Jersey has had public health newborn hearing screening mandated since 1977. Prior to discharge from the hospital, nurses or pediatricians screen all infants for high-risk factors associated with hearing impairment. Parents of the high-risk infants are counseled and provided with pertinent literature. When the infant is 5 months old, the parents receive a letter and a screening report form, which they are instructed to take to their infant's physician. At the time of this writing, the physician is expected to screen the infant for hearing loss; however, the program's directors are studying the need to establish countywide hearing screening centers that would house certified audiologists. These are expected to be operational by October 1, 1985. Once the infant is screened, the physician or center returns the completed form to the program. If the infant passes the screening, his or her name is removed from the hearing risk registry and the parents receive a letter advising them that the infant passed. If the infant fails hearing screening, the parents are sent a second letter recommending hearing follow-up, which may include medical management or comprehensive hearing evaluation or both. A list of audiology centers in the state are provided, which includes a limited number of state funded clinics that provide economic accessibility to audiological services. The physician or audiologist returns the second reporting form to the health department. Again, if the infant passes, his or her name is removed from the hearing risk registry and a letter is sent to the parents. If the infant fails the second evaluation but hearing loss is not confirmed, the infant continues to be followed. When a hearing loss is confirmed, infants are registered with the Special Child Health Services Birth Defects/Service Registry. The parents are informed of other services, including case management, financial assistance for hearing aids, and early intervention. A new data system for the newborn hearing screening program is being devised. No specific data are available at the time of this writing.

Florida

Florida legislation requires that all hospitals complete a high-risk registry for all infants born in the state. As of 1984, 10 hospitals across the state participate, all having perinatal intensive care centers. Auditory brainstem response is used as the initial screening test. Following screening in the hospital, each infant who fails is seen for a complete hearing evaluation. Infants found to be hearing impaired are referred to the Florida Diagnostic Learning Resources System for educational placement and management and to Children's Medical Service for health care. No program data are yet available.

Oklahoma

A statewide program to screen all live births in Oklahoma was implemented in August 1983. The State Department of Health uses a high-risk register as its initial screening procedure to be completed on the approximately 55,000 newborns annually. The risk register form is completed during the infant's stay in the hospital, and families of at-risk infants are contacted when the infant is approximately 4 months old. This mailing recommends that the family have their infant's hearing tested through the agency of their choice. Families not responding receive a second mailing when their child is 6 months old. Limited follow-up audiological services are available and are provided cooperatively through state agencies and private resources. Program goals are to increase availability of follow-up audiological services and initiation of an awareness and training program for hospitals to increase accuracy and compliance in reporting. No data are yet available.

Colorado

In 1977, Colorado Hearing and Speech Services initiated an ''at risk for hearing loss'' segment to its total program. The effort began with a statewide information campaign to the medical community, stressing the importance of early identification and habilitation of infants with serious hearing loss. Testing and habilitation were made available in the child's home community. An informational pamphlet is distributed to the parents of newborns of participating hospitals. The pamphlet outlines expected speech, language, and listening skills for babies from birth to 2 years of age and informs parents that hearing loss may delay a child's speech and language development. It also offers a free hearing test upon request for babies 6 months of age and older. Hospitals throughout Colorado are invited to inform the state program of children at risk according to the Joint Committee's 1982 risk criteria. An estimated 60 percent of Colorado's at-risk children are either being followed by the state or by 10 hospitals with independent high-risk programs. When the at-risk infant is 6 months old, the Department of Health sends a nonalarming letter to the parents that encourages speech and language stimulation, describes behavior that might suggest hearing problems, and again offers a free hearing test for the child. In an effort to improve testing capabilities in outlying areas, a series of portable visual reinforcement audiometry units were built to permit testing in the child's home community by regional audiologists. Babies found with hearing loss are examined by otolaryngologists at local health department otology clinics. Babies with serious hearing loss are registered in the Home Intervention Program, which provides weekly home parental instruction in techniques to stimulate speech, language, and listening skills. According to H. Weber (personal communication, October 22, 1984), from 1977 to 1984, 3,808 children were identified as being at risk, for which 315 hearing tests were requested through the Health Department. Of infants tested, 107 were found to have hearing problems, including 20 with serious sensorineural losses, 8 with mild to moderate sensorineural losses, and 79 with conductive losses.

Arkansas

A unique high-risk hearing screening program is in effect in various hospitals throughout Arkansas involving the Department of Health, the Telephone Pioneers of Central Arkansas, the Optimist Club, and private donations. Volunteers sort hospital completed high-risk forms and inform parents of at-risk infants that a 3-week postnatal auditory brainstem response screening is available for their infant. After screening results are interpreted by an audiologist, the parents are informed by letter. If the infant "fails" or the results are questionable, either a rescreening is performed, a referral is made for more comprehensive testing, or a referral is made to a specialist for examination. Because hospital participation is voluntary, F. Beggs (personal communication, June 16, 1983) reports that there are instances in which high-risk forms are not completed at all or are completed incorrectly. During 1982, 200 infants were identified as being at risk, of which 85 were screened. Of these, two were found to have severe or profound sensorineural losses, and five with possible conductive losses were referred for medical examination. Item analysis of the risk factor occurrence rates follows: maternal rubella = 8.5 percent, family history = 54.5 percent, herpes = 1 percent, premature birth or low birthweight = 3.5 percent, maxillofacial abnormalities = 1 percent, hyperbilirubinemia = 23.5 percent, Apgar scores below 5 at 1 or 5 minutes = 12 percent, and other = 2 percent. On-site testing has recently been added to the program, and regionalization will eventually incorporate approximately 70 percent of all live births in the state.

Nova Scotia

The province of Nova Scotia has a comprehensive high-risk hearing screening program that is simplified by the fact that most live births occur in one major medical facility in the city of Halifax. During the past 6 years, approximately 30,000 live births have been screened by a risk register, which indicates 6 to 7 percent of the newborns were at risk. At-risk infants receive a behavioral screen in the nursery and follow-up through the Nova Scotia Hearing and Speech Clinic, which has 18 regional centers. Public health nurses assist by providing home screening or by encouraging parents to attend secondary screening appointments. The family physician is also notified of the risk condition by letter. The program directors believe that these efforts have been well defined and well managed in that they report an average identification of 1 sensorineural hearing impaired infant per 1,000 live births in the general nursery. In addition, the Province has an effective tertiary intensive care screening program.

California

California law mandates that the State Department of Health, in consultation with participating newborn intensive care centers, establish a system to screen and follow newborns at risk for deafness and establish and maintain quality test protocols. The bill only applies to graduates of those units participating in Crippled Children's Service (CCS) programs. Specific risk criteria, hearing screening, and hearing evaluation protocols have been developed, as have fee schedules that CCS will pay for testing eligible infants. Screening occurs between 3 and 6 months of age, using observation of behavioral or electrophysiological response to sound. Diagnostic procedures include a general physical examination, history and laboratory tests for perinatal infections, and a comprehensive audiological evaluation, including behavioral observation audiometry or auditory evoked potentials if indicated. No specific program data are available.

Wisconsin

Similar to California, the Wisconsin Bureau of Children with Physical Needs will pay agencies to screen and follow up children identified as high risk for a wide variety of disorders at the time of newborn intensive care unit discharge. Testing and follow-up protocols were developed by the Wisconsin Association for Perinatal Care, demonstrating unique public-private agency cooperation. Screening is a comprehensive multifaceted procedure. It includes nursing and interval history; general physical and neurological screen; sensory screening, including vision, hearing, and speech and language development, developmental screening; psychosocial profile; nutritional feeding assessment; analysis; family interpretation; and data collection. No specific patient data were made available at the time of this writing.

Ohio

The Ohio Department of Health has been involved in limited newborn hearing screening since 1968, concentrating initially on Level III newborn intensive care units. It is reported that the program is expanding to all newborns of several hospitals; however, the extent of governmental coordination or follow-up is unclear. The Communicative and Sensory Disorders Unit of the Health Department is requesting mandatory legislation and funding to implement the program in 1985.

Arizona

Arizona has recently formed an interdisciplinary task force to plan statewide early identification and follow-up of children at risk for hearing loss. Professionals have been collaborating to develop protocols that will work within various health care settings. A unique feature of the proposal is the screening by parental questionnaire of 18-month-old children who attend well-baby clinics. Implementation is targeted for the fall of 1985, through the office of Maternal and Child Health, Department of Health Services.

Alaska

Finally, the Alaska Communicative Disorders program has attempted to centralize high-risk hearing screening for a number of years. Due to unique geographic, cultural, and health care delivery problems, a single statewide program to detect sensorineural hearing loss in infancy remains a challenge of the future.

SUMMARY

It has been long realized that early identification of hearing loss is critical to optimal habilitative outcome and that high-risk screening is a sensitive method of identifying deafness at an early age. In spite of this long-term knowledge, these endeavors are just beginning to be implemented on a scale large enough to significantly reduce the morbidity and adverse economic impact of hearing loss in our society. It is apparent that aggressive public health high-risk screening and follow-up programs are prerequisite to significant progress in this vital area.

The major purpose of this chapter is to disseminate information concerning recent progress in governmental large-scale high-risk hearing screening programs in North America. Hopefully, this information will serve to stimulate the growth of new efforts by demonstrating that high-risk hearing screening of large newborn populations is feasible through a variety of programmatic approaches. The ultimate goal is the universal screening of all newborns, as recommended by the Nova Scotia Conference in 1975. Although bureaucratic involvement in innovative projects is an extremely slow process, the growing number of government-sponsored high-risk hearing screening programs suggests an increasing public health commitment toward the early identification of the hearing impaired.

REFERENCES

Altman, M. M. (1968). *Methods of early detection of hearing loss: Final report.* Haifa, Israel: H. Rambam Government Hospital.

Beck, T. (1981). *Infant hearing loss: Statewide screening programs.* Unpublished manuscript. (Available from Deafness Research Foundation, 55 East 34th Street, New York, NY 10016).

Bergstrom, L., Hemenway, W., and Downs, M. (1971). A high-risk registry to find congenital deafness. *Otolaryngology Clinics of North America, 4,* 369–399.

Budetti, P., Barrand, N., McManus, P., and Heiner, L. (1981). *The costs and effectiveness of neonatal intensive care: Case Study #10.* Cost-Effectiveness Analysis of Medical Technology, Office of Technology Assessment. Washington, DC: U.S. Government Printing Office.

Clark, T. (1980, October). *Project SKI*HI newsletter.* Logan: Utah State University.

Downs, D. W. (1982). Auditory brainstem response testing in a neonatal intensive care unit: A cautious response. *ASHA, 24,* 1009–1015.

Ehrlich, C. H., Shapiro, E., Kimball, B. D., and Henther, M. (1973). Communication skills in five-year-old children with high-risk neonatal histories. *Journal of Speech and Hearing Research, 16,* 522–529.

Feinmesser, M., and Tell, L. (1976). Neonatal screening for detection of deafness. *Archives of Otolaryngology, 102,* 297–299.

Feinmesser, M., Tell, L., and Levi, H. (1982). Follow-up of 40,000 infants screened for hearing defect. *Audiology, 21,* 197–203.

Fitch, J. L., Williams, T. F., and Etienne, J. E. (1982). A community-based high-risk register for hearing loss. *Journal of Speech and Hearing Disorders, 47,* 373–375.

FitzZaland, R. E. (1985). Identification of hearing loss in newborns: Results of eight years' experience with a high-risk hearing register. *Volta Review, 87*(4), 195–203.

Galambos, R., Hicks, G. E., and Wilson, M. J. (1982). Identification audiometry in infants: A reply to Simmons. *Ear and Hearing, 3,* 189–190.

Gerber, S. (1976, November). *Conduct and follow-up of a high-risk register.* Paper presented at the annual meeting of American Speech-Language-Hearing Association, Houston.

Green, H. G., Nelson, C. J., Gaylor, D. W., and Holson, J. F. (1979). Accuracy of birth certificate data for detecting facial cleft defects in Arkansas children. *Cleft Palate Journal, 16,* 167–170.

Hirsch, A., and Kankkunen, A. (1974). High-risk history in the identification of hearing loss in newborns. *Scandinavian Audiology, 3,* 177–182.

Lenneberg, E. H. (1967). *Biological Foundations of Language.* New York: John Wiley and Sons.

Loyd, D., and Hankla, J. (1983). *Georgia Southeast Health District Infant High-Risk Hearing Project.* Unpublished manuscript. (Available from Southeast Health Unit, 1101 Church St., Waycross, GA 31501.)

Mahoney, T., and Eichwald, J. (1979). Newborn high-risk hearing screening by maternal questionnaire. *Journal of the American Auditory Society, 5,* 41–45.

Mahoney, T. (1984). High-risk hearing screening of large general newborn populations. *Seminars in Hearing, 5*(1), 25–36.

Marshall, R. E., Reichert, T. J., Kerley, S. M., and Davis, H. (1980). Auditory function in newborn intensive care unit patients revealed by auditory brainstem potentials. *Journal of Pediatrics, 96,* 731–735.

Mencher, G. T. (1974). A program of neonatal screening. *Audiology, 13,* 495–500.

Mencher, G. T. (1975). Nova Scotia conference on the early identification of hearing loss: A review. *Human Communication Journal, 3,* 5–20.

Meyer, D., and Wolfe, V. (1975). Use of a high-risk register in newborn hearing screening. *Journal of Speech and Hearing Disorders, 40,* 493–498.

Northern, J., and Downs, M. (1974). *Hearing in children.* Baltimore: Williams and Wilkins.

Northern, J., and Downs, M. (1978). *Hearing in children* (2nd ed.). Baltimore: Williams and Wilkins.

Salmivalli, A., Suonpaa, J., Johansson, R., and Jauhiainen, T. (1980). Early detection and identification of congenital hearing defects. *Suomen Laakari-lehli, 8.*

Simmons, F. B. (1982). Comment on "Hearing loss in graduates of tertiary intensive care nursery." *Ear and Hearing, 3,* 188.

Stewart, J. (1974). *HRS screening.* Presented at the Western Society for Pediatric Research, Carmel, CA.

Appendix **8–A**

States and Provinces with High-Risk Hearing Screening Programs

States and provinces known to have in operation or to be planning statewide or regional high-risk hearing screening programs and persons to contact.

Alabama (statewide planning)

Supervisor, Speech and Hearing
   Services
Crippled Children's Service
2129 E. So. Boulevard
Montgomery, AL 36199
(205) 288-0220

Alaska (statewide planning)

Director, Speech and Hearing
3401 East 42nd Avenue
Anchorage, AK 99504
(907) 562-2675

Arizona (statewide planning)

Manager, Hearing Conservation
   Program
Maternal and Child Health Services
200 North Curry Road
Tempe, AZ 85281
(602) 968-6461

Arkansas (regional active)

Director, Speech and Hearing
   Services
State Department of Health
4815 West Markham
Little Rock, AR 72201
(501) 661-2328

British Columbia (province active)

Director, Speech and Hearing
Rotherham Place
1520 Blanshard St., 3rd Floor
Victoria, BC Canada V8W 3C8
(604) 387-1575

California (statewide planning)

Hearing Conservation Specialist
Maternal and Child Health Branch
Department of Health Services
714 P Street
Sacramento, CA 95814
(916) 322-2950

Colorado (statewide active)

Chief, Hearing and Speech Services
Handicapped Children's Program
Colorado Department of Health
4210 East 11th Avenue
Denver, CO 80220
(303) 320-6137

Connecticut (statewide planning)

Director, Speech Pathology and
   Audiology
Connecticut State Department of
   Health
Health Services for Handicapped
   Children's Section
79 Elm Street
Hartford, CT 06115
(203) 566-4344

Florida (regional active)

Chief, Audiology
University of Florida
Gainesville, FL 32601
(904) 392-2636

Adapted from Mahoney (1984)

Georgia (regional active)

Director
Child-Adolescent Health Program
2nd Floor, Family Health Section
878 Peach Tree Street, NE
Atlanta, GA 30309
(404) 656-4830

Maryland (statewide planning)

Director
Speech Pathology and Audiology
State Department of Health and
    Mental Hygiene
201 West Preston Street
Baltimore, MD 21201
(301) 383-2847

Massachusetts (statewide active)

Coordinator, Hearing and Vision
    Services
Department of Public Health
Maternal and Child Health
80 Boylston Street
Boston, MA 02116
(617) 727-0941

New Jersey (statewide active)

Speech Pathology/Audiology
    Consultant
Special Child Health Services
Department of Health
120 So. Stockton Street CN 364
Trenton, NJ 08625

Nova Scotia (province active)

Director
Nova Scotia Hearing and Speech
    Clinic
Fenwick Place
5599 Fenwick Street
Halifax, Nova Scotia, Canada B3H
    1R2
(902) 423-7354

Ohio (statewide planning)

Chief
Communicative and Sensory
    Disorders
Ohio Department of Health
Box 118
Columbus, OH 43216
(614) 566-3569

Oklahoma (statewide active)

Director, Pediatric Division
Maternal and Child Health
Oklahoma State Department of
    Health
1000 N. E. 10th
P.O. Box 53551
Oklahoma City, OK 73152
(405) 271-4477
Supervisor
Speech and Hearing Unit
Oklahoma Department of Human
    Services
P.O. Box 25352
Oklahoma City, OK 73125
(405) 521-3589

Rhode Island (statewide planning)

Hearing and Speech Consultant
Division of Child Health and
    Crippled Children's Services
Canyon Health bldg.—Room 302
75 Davis Street
Providence, RI 02908
(401) 277-5040 or 277-5485

Tennessee (statewide active)

Regional Director
Speech and Hearing Services
Department of Health and
    Environment
100 9th Avenue N.
Nashville, TN 37219-5405
(615) 741-7335

Utah (statewide active)

Director
Bureau of Communicative Disorders
Utah Department of Health
44 Medical Drive
Salt Lake City, UT 84113
(801) 533-6175

Wisconsin (statewide planning)

Hearing Consultant
Hearing Conservation Program
Bureau of Children with Physical
  Needs
Department of Public Instruction
125 So. Webster Street
Madison, WI 53702
(608) 266-3890 or 267-9188

SECTION II
MODEL PROGRAMS

Chapter 9

MODEL PROGRAM I
The Crib-o-gram

Children's Hospital
Oakland, California

Adeline Clingan McClatchie
Danielle M. Mikulich

The intensive care nursery (ICN) at Children's Hospital, Oakland, California, is a Level III 40-bed unit that provides comprehensive evaluation and treatment to neonates. These babies, who exhibit a variety of medical and surgical problems and require one-on-one nursing, are transported by aircraft or ambulance from hospitals throughout Northern California to the ICN. The average stay in the nursery is 21 days; however, some babies have an extended sojourn of up to 1 year. The ICN services include a multidisciplinary team consisting of neonatologists, specialized nurses, infant developmentalists, infant psychologists, infant educators, and medical and paramedical personnel who provide quality management. With the low infant mortality rate, the surviving population presents a challenge medically and educationally both in the nursery and in the ensuing years of development. Arising from this challenge is the neonatal follow-up program, providing medical and developmental management and services to children with developmental delays and neurological and respiratory problems. Specialty services such as hearing and speech provide an important adjunct.

The Conference on Newborn Hearing Screening (San Francisco, February 1971) invited national involvement, both research and clinical, to assist in finding hearing-impaired infants early for habilitative purposes. Recommendation IX of the proceedings of this conference called for ''validation of the Crib-o-gram approach on a large sample in several institutions with appropriate follow-up.'' This call for research efforts to design screening programs for infants at risk for hearing loss resulted in a pilot hearing screening program being initiated in the ICN in Children's Hospital, Oakland. The majority of babies in the ICN met one or more of the high-risk conditions suggested by the 1971 Joint Committee on Newborn Hearing Screening. Those babies who did not meet these criteria were still included in the hearing screening program, because they were present in the nursery.

DEVELOPMENT OF THE PROGRAM

The Center for Childrens' Communication Disorders (CCCD) at Children's Hospital, Oakland, realized the need to screen these ICN babies for potential hearing loss and embarked upon a program using auditory brainstem response (ABR) audiometry in 1977. At that time, the selection of babies for ABR testing was made by the individual physician attending each infant. Referral, therefore, for ABR testing was inconsistent and appeared to be dependent upon the individual physician's knowledge and interest in the field of deafness.

Follow-up of ICN graduates through neonatal follow-up programs in the hospital and in the community medical practices led to suspicion of hearing loss at age 6 to 9 months in some babies not previously referred for ABR testing while in the nursery. The audiology staff, aware of the value of screening while the baby was still in the hospital, sought a simple procedure for hearing screening that would be acceptable to all medical staff and began a search in 1979 for the appropriate screening tool. Although the hospital had available ABR testing, the system was not portable, and audiology personnel could not be made available to test every ICN resident. Therefore, ABR as a screening technique was rejected by a medical committee because it was too expensive and too cumbersome. Crib-o-gram met with greater appeal in medical committees because of its nonintrusiveness and its low cost application.

The full-scale infant hearing screening program using Crib-o-gram as a prerequisite screening for discharge was initiated in 1980. Because Crib-o-gram was a relatively new procedure at that time, with limited supporting statistics, all babies failing Crib-o-gram (50 scalar or below) received ABR testing immediately or within a few days of Crib-o-gram failure. ABR testing was intended to define the nature of the failing baby's hearing condition. In an attempt to identify false-negative Crib-o-gram results (passing Crib-o-gram scores for babies actually having a hearing loss), every fifth baby who passed a Crib-o-gram screen also received ABR testing.

The test results of the first 120 babies screened with Crib-o-gram were reviewed. There was a 16 percent failure rate. Of those who failed Crib-o-gram, 60 percent also failed ABR at 70/30 dB HTL screening levels.

Many babies failing Crib-o-gram and ABR in the nursery, given time for neurological and developmental maturation, are able to pass ABR at 2 months of age. Therefore, immediate ABR testing for Crib-o-gram failures was discontinued, and all babies failing Crib-o-gram were returned for ABR testing at corrected age of 2 months. Appointment time for ABR testing was provided at the time of discharge.

Every fifth baby who passed Crib-o-gram also passed ABR testing. Therefore, the procedure of ABR testing for every fifth baby who passed Crib-o-gram was discontinued, because no significant difference between the two procedures was recorded to substantiate further investigation.

Follow-up protocol revealed a small number of babies who had Crib-o-gram scores between 50 and 59, with hearing impairment of a mild degree as determined by later ABR testing. Consequently, the "passing scalar score" was raised from 50 to 60 at this institution. Since 1982, only one baby, for whom there was no etiology or medical condition indicative of a progressive hearing loss, had a scalar score greater than 60 and was later identified with a moderate hearing loss.

SCREENING PROTOCOL

Volunteers

In 1982, a volunteer program was initiated with a team of three volunteers who provided screening services to the nursery three times per week. Babies discharged between these volunteer testing times were screened by their nurses. It is mandatory that the individual receive training in administering the test and recording the results by the managing audiologist. The procedures involved in scrubbing, swabbing the instrument, setting up the Crib-o-gram, calibrating it, and documenting the results are kept in writing beside the instrument to assist easy recall. Standardization of all procedures is necessary to obtain reliable results. The individual who is screening the baby is responsible for recording and reporting scalar scores on the appropriate form (Appendix 9–A). The forms are sent to CCCD, and results are written in the infant's medical chart to alert the attending physician.

Procedures

The screening protocol is outlined in Table 9–1. An explanation of Crib-o-gram screening is provided in writing for all parents (Appen-

TABLE 9–1. Intensive Care Nursery Auditory Screening Flow Chart Used at Children's Hospital

In nursery 2–3 days prior to discharge	2 Crib-o-grams	
	FAIL: 59 scalar or less	**PASS:** Neonatal follow-up medical program
	Registered letter to managing pediatrician	Behavioral audiological and acoustic impedance at 9–12 months at CCCD
Return to CCCD 2 months after discharge	ABR Impedance	
	FAIL	
Within 1 month of ABR	Behavioral audiometry Impedance	
	FAIL	
Immediately following	Information shared with parent, physician, financing agency	
	Medical clearance for hearing aid	
Within 4 weeks of behavioral audiometry	Hearing aid testing, fitting, and parent counseling	
Immediately following	Enrolled in infant–parent program for hearing impaired at CCCD	
When appropriate	Relevant school placement	
Biannual	Follow-up audiological testing	

dix 9–B). Every baby in the intensive care nursery is given two Crib-o-gram screens. A scalar score of less than 60 either time results in referral for ABR testing at 2 months of age. At the time of discharge, those babies who fail the Crib-o-gram screening are given an appointment for a return visit to the audiology department in approximately 2 months. A registered letter indicating the screening failure is forwarded to the managing physician, with a reminder of the follow-up requirements (Appendix 9–C). Potential funding agencies for initial hearing testing are also informed. Many infants seen at the hospital come from outlying areas, and return is difficult. Selecting an alternate facility to perform hearing testing is the responsibility of the physician managing the baby.

Reports of ABR testing at 2 months post-nursery discharge are sent to the baby's managing physician, nursery physician, and other specialists who may be involved with the child's care, including the funding agency. Audiological recommendations are made pertaining to further audiological management and follow-up.

Consideration of amplification is begun immediately if testing indicates significant hearing loss. If the managing physician is in agreement, habilitation is available for the family and child at CCCD in conjunction with hearing aid selection. In the event that hearing is eventually found within normal limits but poor listening and auditory skills are seen or reported, a therapeutic program is designed to assist parents in ways of stimulating good listening behavior.

The neonatal medical follow-up program provides home and clinic-based developmental follow-up for the majority of the ICN graduates. Pediatric examinations are scheduled at 3- to 6-month intervals during the first 2 years of life. Care is coordinated with family pediatricians, community agencies, and other professionals to ensure that the infant's and family's needs are met. Protocol within this program requires audiological review of all intensive care graduates at 9 to 12 months. This consists of extended behavioral testing with headphones and acoustic impedance measurement. This protocol is helpful in finding those babies who failed Crib-o-gram and who have not returned for follow-up testing. It also ensures that those babies who pass Crib-o-gram screening but have high-risk etiologies, medical conditions, or medical treatments aligned with progressive auditory problems are audiologically reviewed on a longitudinal basis.

Long-stay babies who have developed beyond the reflexive responsive level to sound receive ABR testing when they are sufficiently stable. They are followed audiologically in the nursery with intervention when it is considered appropriate to the baby's overall well-being. An example is an infant who manifests major conductive hearing loss as a sequel to a congenital syndrome with partial or total absence of middle ear ossicles (Nager's syndrome). If these long-stay babies are emotionally and interactively ready, they are provided with amplification in the nursery under careful supervision. In contrast, others have not been given amplification until close to discharge time, because their conditions reflected limited ability to handle additional stimulation in the busy ICN environment.

RESULTS

As described in this chapter, Crib-o-gram screening is presently accepted at Children's Hospital, Oakland as an alternative to the high-risk register for referring infants in the intensive care nursery for more extensive hearing testing. A summary of hearing losses detected through the hearing screening program is illustrated in Table 9–2. During the 5 years of investigating Crib-o-gram screening in an

TABLE 9–2. Incidence of Screening Failure and Confirmed Hearing Loss at the Children's Hospital, Oakland

Year	1980	1981	1982	1983	1984	Total
Total screened	210	276	243	340	293	1362
Number failed—Scalar 50	33	40	44	50	50	217
Number failed—Scalar 50–59	N/A	N/A	11	33	35	79
Percent total failed—60	N/A	N/A	22.6	24.4	29.0	21.7
Percent of total screened with sensorineural loss	2.4	1.4	2.4	2.9	7.1	3.4
Degree of bilateral sensorineural loss						
Profound	1	1	1	0	2	5
Severe	1	1	1	1	3*	7
Moderate	1	1	3	4 + 1*	6 + 1*	17
Mild	2	0	1	1	6	10
High-frequence	0	1	0	1	1	3
Progressive	0	0	0	2	2*	4
Total sensorineural loss	5	4	6	10	21	46
Percent of Crib-o-gram fail with sensorineural loss	15.1	10.0	10.9	12.0	24.7	15.5
Additional hearing losses identified but not included above						
Conductive	N/A	2	1	0	2	5
Unilateral sensorineural	1	1	3	3	2	10

*No Crib-o-gram screen because of severity of condition of long-stay nursery residents. Hearing loss confirmed later by BSERA.

intensive care nursery, 46 babies of the 1362 screened have documented bilateral sensorineural hearing losses significant for amplification. Another five babies have documented conductive losses pertaining to syndromes and require extensive medical management paralleling audiological management. Despite the fact that Crib-o-gram is a sound field stimulus and not ear specific, in this 5-year period, 10 unilateral sensorineural hearing losses have been found in the Crib-o-gram failure group. One baby passed Crib-o-gram with later follow-up indicating hearing problems. This baby has had failure to thrive and has been returned to Children's Hospital with multiple medical problems. It is possible that the hearing loss had been progressive; however, no significant medical findings to date support this premise.

The long-stay ICN baby continues to present difficulties in audiological management and inclusion in studies of screening effectiveness. Often not included in Crib-o-gram studies because of the state of the baby at the appropriate time for testing, the infant is later referred for ABR. In 1984, three babies were found with severe to profound hearing losses in this group with no Crib-o-gram screening (note asterisks in 1984 column). One other baby was diagnosed with moderately severe sensorineural hearing loss. These babies are included in the total number in Table 9–2, so hearing loss is not overlooked in the final count. As of this writing, 28 percent of 1984 babies have yet to return for the 2-month follow-up.

DISCUSSION

A high-risk register had not been used effectively by physicians in the referral process for ABR hearing screening in this institution. This ineffectiveness led to the introduction and development of the Crib-o-gram protocol described earlier in this chapter.

In using Crib-o-gram screening, approximately one fourth of the total ICN population is referred for further audiological review. In 1984, one of four Crib-o-gram failures manifested hearing loss requiring audiological management. At this center, Crib-o-gram provides a more cost-effective screening than ABR for every ICN baby. The cost for Crib-o-gram screening is approximately $22 per baby and is less than one third the cost of ABR screening. The percent of referral for further testing is typically higher for Crib-o-gram screening than for ABR screening. This increases the cost of the follow-up program. Nevertheless, the total cost of screening and follow-up is estimated to be lower with Crib-o-gram screening than with ABR screening in the ICN at this institution.

The delay of 2 months for follow-up ABR testing, as opposed to immediate testing following a Crib-o-gram failure, appears effective in identifying babies with a hearing loss and reducing the cost of the screening procedures.

The neonatal follow-up program for babies leaving the ICN provides a relatively consistent check on those babies who have passed Crib-o-gram while in intensive care. Any baby failing to meet the behavioral extended screening at 9 months to 1 year of age is referred for comprehensive audiological testing, which includes ABR and acoustic impedance audiometry.

Has Crib-o-gram screening been effective? When this center relied on the use of the high-risk register, a random selection of infants were seen for ABR testing and audiological follow-up. Crib-o-gram now serves as a screening device for all ICN babies. It is noninvasive, cost-effective, and low in personnel requirements. In conjunction with a neonatal follow-up medical program, Crib-o-gram has been an effective tool for identification of infants with potential hearing impairment.

Crib-o-gram screening cannot be viewed as a program by itself in an ICN. To be effective, it must interface with a follow-up audiological and medical program. Used as a general indicator of babies requiring further auditory testing, Crib-o-gram screening can play an effective role in the early identification of hearing loss.

Appendix **9–A**

Form for Recording Hearing Screening Results

DATA COLLECTION # _____________   (Use space to imprint patient name, Data Processing #, PF #, and other admissions information.)

CENTER FOR CHILDREN'S
COMMUNICATION DISORDERS
Children's Hospital Medical Center
51st and Grove Streets
Oakland, CA 94609

AUDITORY SCREENING AND TESTING REFERRAL

Child's Physician (for continuing care): __________________________
                                          (Name)

____
(Address)

____

(Phone)

Attending House Physician: __________________________
                            (Name)
____

CRIB-O-GRAM DATA: Date:___________   ON: ________
               Performed by: _______   OFF: ________
Primary Diagnosis: ______________________________________
Secondary Diagnosis: ____________________________________
RESULTS: SCALAR NUMBER: ___________
               PASS ☐   REFER ☐   (Check One)

	(Circle)	
Child is part of interaction program (CDC).	Yes	No
Billing slip has been stamped and attached.	Yes	No
Crib-o-gram information (pink copy) has been placed in chart.	Yes	No
Failure has been phoned to CCCD.	Yes	No

Appendix 9–B

Explanation of Hearing Loss for Parents of Intensive Care Nursery Babies

Babies learn very important things about their environment and about communication through their ears in the first 12 months of life. This is the time when a baby learns through cooing and babbling the beginning of speech sounds. Early detection of a hearing loss in early infancy helps both the baby and the family to make the best possible adjustment. Babies can develop hearing loss from any of the factors documented in the at-risk category for hearing impairment (a copy of this is enclosed). These factors can result in damage to the nerve of hearing. Damage can be partial or severe. The degree can be documented in the hearing testing. If the baby has a mild hearing loss, his language and speech can develop normally. If a moderate or severe hearing loss is found, the baby may require the use of hearing aids. Specialists are available through audiology and speech clinics to assist families in understanding the use of hearing aids and to direct their learning about hearing loss and language and speech development. The development of speech occurs during the first 3 years of life.

Hearing screening can be carried out in many ways. Screening means sorting out those babies who require further testing to find out whether hearing is normal or not. Crib-o-gram, as we use in our nursery, is a computerized form of hearing screening. Hearing testing can be carried out at birth but has better validity at 2 months of age in the premature baby. Brainstem Evoked Response Audiometry is a test using electrodes and headphones. The baby's responses are obtained by computer averaging of miniscule responses within the brain to certain sound stimuli. Thousands of these responses are averaged and recorded. The test is given while the baby is asleep.

Remember that hearing screening is a safeguard for your baby. If your baby needs further testing, please be sure that you keep appointments. Some people think that it does not matter if their baby does not hear well during the first year. This is not true. For speech to develop, a baby must be aware of sound early.

If you have any questions regarding hearing loss in infancy or about treatment of hearing loss, please call the Center for Children's Communication Disorders.

Yours sincerely,

Audiology Staff
Center for Children's Communication
Disorders

Appendix **9–C**

Letter to Baby's Physician Explaining Screening Failure

Date:

Re:
D.O.B.:
CHMC Nursery Discharge:

Dear Dr. ___________________ :

This baby was included in our routine auditory screening procedure and failed to meet screening criteria. It is important that the baby is referred for audiological follow-up, because there is high risk of some degree of hearing loss.

Appointment for a Brainstem Evoked Response Audiometry test has been set for ______________________ as our recommended follow-up procedure. In the event that the family fail to show for this appointment (which will be confirmed 24 hours before by CCCD) or cancel the appointment, the audiological program at CHMC will assume the case to be closed until further contact by the physician in charge of care. Notation of *no show* will be mailed to your office.

A report of BSERA findings will be sent to you following the procedure.

If you refer the baby to California Children's Service, the cost of service can be covered by that agency. Thank you for your attention to referral and follow-up.

Sincerely,

Coordinator Audiological Services   Director, Regional Newborn
                                                Intensive Care Program

cc: CCS

Chapter **10**

MODEL PROGRAM II
A High-Risk Register and Auditory Brainstem Response

Children's Hospital of Pittsburgh
Pittsburgh, Pennsylvania

Kathi E. Kurmin
Thomas J. Fria

PROGRAM SETTING

The audiology department of Children's Hospital located in metropolitan Pittsburgh has conducted hearing screening for newborns 5 days per week since 1981. These audiology services are provided on a contractual basis between Children's Hospital and other hospitals in the Pittsburgh area. The majority of newborns are screened at Magee Women's Hospital, where approximately 10,000 births occur each year.

PROGRAM DEVELOPMENT

Using the auditory brainstem response (ABR) in screening entails much more than buying the latest equipment and then commencing with a barrage of screening tests. The likelihood of a program's success is greatly enhanced when careful attention is paid to a series of prerequisite activities. A series of activities predated the newborn screening program at Children's Hospital of Pittsburgh. A description of the screening program itself will be given below, but first it is important to highlight the activities that preceded the onset of testing.

Determination of Costs

Although the thought of cost in a screening program may seem callous, these aspects must eventually be addressed. We found it helpful to have a firm grasp of just what the program would cost and how that cost would be covered when dealing with administrative officials. Considerations in determining the costs were discussed in an earlier publication by Fria (1985) and are reproduced here:

> There are three main cost aspects: equipment, personnel, and indirect expenses. These costs must be considered in the context of the number of babies you intend to screen over a given period of time, usually one year. If we assume that an ABR system typically costs $20,000 and we would like to earn this money back in the first five years of operation, then $4000 in direct equipment expense is estimated in each of the first five years. In addition, the equipment must then be depreciated typically over a period of five years. In other words, one fifth of the cost of the equipment ($4000) must be assigned to each of the first five years of operation so that a new device can be purchased when the present one wears out! Therefore, the total cost of equipment in this hypothetical situation is $8000 per year.
>
> The cost of personnel must then be estimated. Let's say that we plan to have a person spend 20 hours a week (approximately "half time") conducting the tests and coordinating the program. If this person is paid $12,300 (including 23 percent fringe benefits) then this figure must be added to the total cost per year. This brings the total to $20,300, including equipment and personnel.
>
> Indirect costs also enter into the picture. These expenses are attributed to the cost of running the hospital, such as salaries of people who do not see patients (administration, housekeeping, maintenance, etc.) and miscellaneous expenses such as utilities. Usually these expenses are estimated at 25 percent of the direct cost (equipment and personnel). Consequently, we have to include 25 percent of $20,300, or approximately $5000, to our total. Finally, we have to add one more indirect cost which is sometimes called a "bad debt" allowance. This is the cost of not collecting all the money owed to the hospital and is usually estimated as an additional 25 percent.
>
> Therefore, the total screening program costs will be approximately $30,300. The cost per test, then, would equal this amount divided by the number of anticipated ABR screening tests in one year. For example, if 500 tests are anticipated then the cost per test would be approximately $60. If, however, only 100 tests are planned, the cost per test will increase dramatically. Consequently, the cost per infant may realistically preclude using the ABR at your facility unless a fairly large number of babies require screening, or the program can be subsidized in other ways.

Preliminary Contacts

In addition to administrative officials, it was also important to contact the medical personnel who have a vested interest in the planned screening. Included in this group were neonatologists, pediatricians, and nursing supervisors. These people were informed of the screening program and specific plans to carry it out. Neonatologists and pediatricians were informed about congenital hearing loss, high-risk factors, alternative screening procedures, and our specific plans. The nursing supervisor was also given the same information and, in addition, learned what role he or she would play in the program.

These preliminary contacts served to inform professionals of provisions for diagnosis for those babies who failed the screen—exactly where, when, and how often all the high-risk newborns would be followed.

Collection of Normative Data

After preliminary approval to proceed with screening, the first activity was to collect our own sample of ABR data on newborns. The main objective was to determine the minimum stimulus intensity at which all the term newborns yielded an ABR. We were not interested in interwave latency data as much as determining minimal response levels for screening purposes. At this stage, it was also possible to detect problems (i.e., influence of electrical artifact or electrical ground problems) and take corrective action. It was also possible to modify the screening protocol following the collection of the control sample data. This related to type of stimulus, stimulus level, presentation rate, type of electrodes, and earphone arrangement.

Primary Care Physicians and Parents

We discussed the intended screening with the primary care physicians in the community. This gave the physicians a chance to point out practical and philosophical objections to the intended protocols, thereby avoiding unnecessary confrontations in the future. It also provided the opportunity to initiate confidence in the results of the ABR screen. Primary care physicians also had opinions about what parents should be told and how referrals for diagnosis should be made. Following these sessions, the intended follow-up protocol required modification.

Because the nature and extent of interactions with parents are vital to any screening endeavor, we developed two informative pamphlets. One describes the screening program, and the other discusses the development of audition in the infant. These pamphlets consequently serve to describe the tests the newborn may receive and to increase maternal awareness of what to expect of the developing infant during the early months of life. Following approval by hospital officials, these pamphlets were easily distributed to each expectant mother upon admission to the hospital.

We also decided what to "tell" the parents when the ABR test was completed. The reader is referred to an excellent treatment of this important area by Stein and Jabaley (1981). The parents of babies who fail the screen would never be told that the infant had a "hearing loss." They would be told that there were a number of reasons why the baby may not have responded and that the results only mean that it is necessary to conduct further tests when the baby is older. We instructed all the nursery staff, including attending physicians, exactly what the screening results mean. We also found that preprinted cards with a clear explanation of the meaning of the ABR results can be distributed to incoming residents and fellows to counteract any potential misunderstandings.

Logistical Considerations

The logistics of screening with the ABR included a place to store the ABR system when not in use, sterilization of the equipment during use, and a complete safety check of the device by the appropriate hospital personnel.

We also determined the best test time, who would be the primary nursing contact, and how the screening results would be charted. It was important to determine how a charge for the ABR test would be generated and who in the accounting office would facilitate processing.

SCREENING PROGRAM

Neonates born at any hospital under contract with Children's Hospital are reviewed for high-risk criteria contributing to hearing loss. The specific criteria considered are those seven categories suggested by the Joint Committee on Infant Hearing (1982) plus sepsis and neurologic insults (i.e., interventricular bleeding). The complete high-risk register used at this hospital is reproduced in Table 10–1.

The majority of infants at risk come from the intensive care nurseries (ICNs). Infants from the well-baby nurseries can be screened upon referral from the nursing staff or the attending physician or upon parental request. Infants can also be referred from other hospitals in the local area, and these are screened on an outpatient basis.

TEST PROTOCOL

At Magee Women's Hospital, graduates of ICNs are placed in convalescent nurseries prior to being discharged from the hospital.

TABLE 10–1. High-Risk Register Used at Children's Hospital in Pittsburgh

A family history of childhood hearing impairment
Congenital perinatal infection
Anatomical malformations involving the head or neck
Birthweight less than 1500 gm
Hyperbilirubinemia at level exceeding indications for exchange transfusion
Bacterial meningitis
Severe asphyxia
Sepsis
Neurological insult

Here, the infants are in open cribs and detached from monitoring equipment. ABR screening is conducted with a small portable ABR unit (Caldwell, Model 5200) in the afternoon following feeding. Newborns range in age from 34 to 50 weeks post-conception (gestational age plus chronological age).

Both ears are tested with click stimuli at 35 and 70 dB nHL. Based on test results, the infants are listed in one of three categories: pass, fail, and observe. Table 10–2 lists the criteria for inclusion in each of these categories as well as the follow-up protocol.

A click-elicited response in both ears at 35 dB nHL is required for a "pass." "Failure" is a lack of response at 70 dB nHL in one or both ears. Infants who do not yield a repeatable ABR at 35 dB nHL only in both ears are assigned to an "observe" group, because our early experience demonstrated almost universal overreferral upon subsequent retest.

Screening results are reported in the hospital chart and are sent to the primary care physician who is asked to encourage parents to schedule their child for a retest when indicated. To increase follow-up compliance, an appointment card is also placed in the chart at the time of the screening, and this is given to the parents at the time of discharge.

Follow-up behavioral audiometry and repeat ABR tests are given approximately 3 months post-discharge for newborns who fail the screen or who are in the observe category. Because of the high incidence of overreferrals in the latter group, much more emphasis is placed on follow-up tests for the clear failures. If the infant passes both behavioral and ABR tests at 3 months, the parents are requested to return between 6 and 12 months for a behavioral check to monitor development of appropriate auditory behavior. If an infant who originally failed again fails either ABR or behavioral testing at 3 months, habilitation is discussed with the parents and the infant is recalled in the near future to begin habilitative procedures. If an infant was originally in the observe category and again failed either ABR or behavioral testing at 3 months, he or she is referred for medical

TABLE 10–2. Screening and Follow-Up Protocol

	Screening of High-Risk Neonates		
	Pass	*Fail*	*Observe*
Prior to hospital discharge	Response at 35 and 70 dB nHL in both ears	No response at 70 dB nHL in one or both ears	No response in one or both ears at 35 dB nHL with a response at 70 dB nHL in both ears
At 3 months		ABR and Behavioral tests *Fail* *Pass* Start habilitation at next appointment	ABR and Behavioral tests *Fail* *Pass* Referred to pediatrician for medical examination
At 6 months	Behavioral test	Behavioral test	

management, and a request is made for audiological re-evaluation after medical management. The parents of newborns who pass the screen are encouraged to return in 6 months to check for age-appropriate development of auditory behavior.

The charges for screening are based on equipment, personnel, and volume of tests. At present, a charge of approximately $85 per child is necessary to cover costs of the screening program. Reimbursement for screening and follow-up comes through private insurance and funds from the State Department of Health and Department of Public Assistance.

RESULTS

In the early years of the program, approximately 13 percent of newborns failed the ABR screen, and this was evenly divided between clear failures at the highest stimulus intensity and the observe group. Today, we find that approximately 10 percent of the babies fail, but the split is no longer even; the proportion of observes has remained essentially unchanged at 6 to 7 percent, but the percent who fail at 70 dB nHL has dropped by around one half to 3 to 4 percent. At present, we have no clear explanation for this phenomenon. Under the screening program at Children's Hospital, 50 hearing-impaired children have been identified in the 4 years that the program has been running.

SUMMARY

It should be apparent from the above discussion that a substantial amount of work preceded the first ABR screening test. Of course, the test of a successful program should be the number of hearing-impaired infants who have been identified and helped and who might otherwise have gone undetected. The identification of 50 children in 4 years through the screening efforts at Children's Hospital of Pittsburgh seems a significant number. ABR has served as a valuable tool in screening newborns for congenital hearing loss at this hospital.

REFERENCES

Fria, T. J. (1985). Identification of congenital hearing loss with the auditory brainstem response. In J. T. Jacobson (Ed.), *The auditory brainstem response* (pp. 317–334). San Diego: College-Hill Press.

Joint Committee on Infant Hearing (1982). Position statement. *Pediatrics,* 70(3), 496–497.

Stein, L. K., and Jabaley, T. J. (1981). Early identification and parent counseling. In L. K. Stein, E. D. Mindel, and T. J. Jabaley (Eds.), *Deafness and mental health*. New York: Grune and Stratton.

Chapter 11

MODEL PROGRAM III
A High-Risk Register, Behavioral Observation Audiometry, and Auditory Brainstem Response

Northwestern Perinatal Center
Prentice Women's Hospital and Maternity Center
Chicago, Illinois

Wynnette J. Moneka

INTRODUCTION AND PROGRAM SETTING

Prentice Women's Hospital and Maternity Center houses the Northwestern Perinatal Center, one of nine perinatal centers in metropolitan Chicago with neonatal intensive care units (NICU). There are an average of 3,600 live births per year at the maternity center. The 32-bed NICU and the flexible-sized transitional nursery serve approximately 500 babies each year with an average stay of 21 days, while providing all types of nonsurgical care for critically ill infants. This maternity hospital is also the only designated high-risk maternity center in the city; thus, a higher relative proportion of births at this center requires intensive nursery care. About 20 percent of the babies cared for each year are accepted from other hospitals designated as transport sites as part of a four-state regional perinatal network. Of the nine perinatal centers in the area, one other center is known to have a systematic audiology screening program.

INITIAL AUDIOLOGY PROGRAM ORGANIZATION

The audiology screening program has been in effect at Prentice Women's Hospital and Maternity Center since 1977, shortly after the hospital opened. Prior to this, obstetrical and nursery care were provided in two separate hospital pavilions. The building of a centralized maternity hospital allowed for a consolidated effort by the audiology department and, thus, was the motivating factor in initiating the program. Audiology services at the hospital, a multipavilion complex, are on a contractual basis between the hospital and Northwestern University Medical School Audiology and Hearing Impairment Program. During the initial 18 months, the screening program was established and operated through an informal arrangement. The neonatologists were asked to share their reactions to the provision of this new service and indicate whether or not they thought it should be an ongoing service. The audiology department also evaluated the program for the over-all time required, the efficiency of the screenings as judged by pass-fail ratios, and habilitative demands. During this evaluative period, no fees were charged for the testing, and, thus, for medical-legal reasons, the results were not recorded in the medical chart by the audiologist. Rather, all hearing screening results were forwarded to the neonatologists, who, at their discretion, could report or file them in the infant's outpatient chart.

CURRENT PROGRAM ORGANIZATION

After the first 18 months of the screening program, the audiology department combined efforts with those of a group of associated professionals, and, since that time, services have been rendered through a hospital-based developmental evaluation clinic (DEC). The individual team members represent developmental psychology, neonatology, ophthamology, parent-infant education, physical therapy, speech pathology, and audiology. The decision to combine professional efforts for follow-up care was made because of the generalized risk status of many infants. At this center, six items are slated as mutual factors for both audiological and developmental services:

1. Birthweight of 1500 gm or less
2. Five-minnute Apgar score of five or less, or other indications of significant asphyxia
3. Intrauterine viral or nonbacterial infections (i.e., TORCH infections)
4. Bacterial meningitis
5. Cranial defects, including trisomy 21, but excluding isolated cleft lip or palate

6. Other indices of suspicion: significant visual defects, seizures, metabolic acidosis, adoptive status, or genetic disease known to be associated with developmental or sensory impairments

Four additional factors are included in the audiology-only protocol:

1. Bilirubin of a level high enough to require treatment for more than 3 days by phototherapy, or any transfused baby
2. Positive family history of hearing loss
3. Ototoxic medications administered for more than 3 days
4. Cranial or facial defects in isolation

The risk factors listed above have been in use since 1978 and are more comprehensive than those of the 1982 Position Statement of the Joint Committee on Infant Hearing. Continued use of items in addition to the Joint Committee's list resulted from programmatic experience with identified cases of hearing loss in which ototoxic medications and hyperbilirubinemia were prevalent items (Moneka and Gollegly, 1983).

Following the merger with these other professional services, the audiology program targeted three ages for routine audiological evaluations: prior to discharge from the nursery, 9 to 12 months of age, and 2½ to 3½ years of age. The age-related goals and test protocols were defined to fit the levels of development so that particular degrees and types of hearing loss could be identified. The establishment of target ages also permitted identification of team-related goals for these ages.

Figure 11–1 illustrates the organization of the audiology program across ages. On this figure, "routine" follow-up refers to the recommended services a child would receive if he or she passed the test criteria at each specified age level. This "routine" track progressively rules out lesser degrees of hearing loss as the child matures and completes additional behavioral and impedance audiometry tests.

Tables 11–1, 11–2, and 11–3 provide the specific audiological protocols and goals for the "routine" audiology track by age level. The non-audiological goals, listed as supplemental medical and developmental goals for each age, evolved as part of the team concept for management of this population. Specifying these goals encourages the standardized formulation of recommendations and management plans for each child.

In Figure 11–1, "non-routine" follow-up care refers to children who do not pass the specified audiological criteria or those confirmed to have a hearing impairment. Individualized follow-up of these cases would include auditory brainstem response (ABR) testing as a supplemental test whenever warranted, and these cases would be seen as often as is audiologically or medically necessary. At the nursery screening level, note that the "non-routine" track is based not

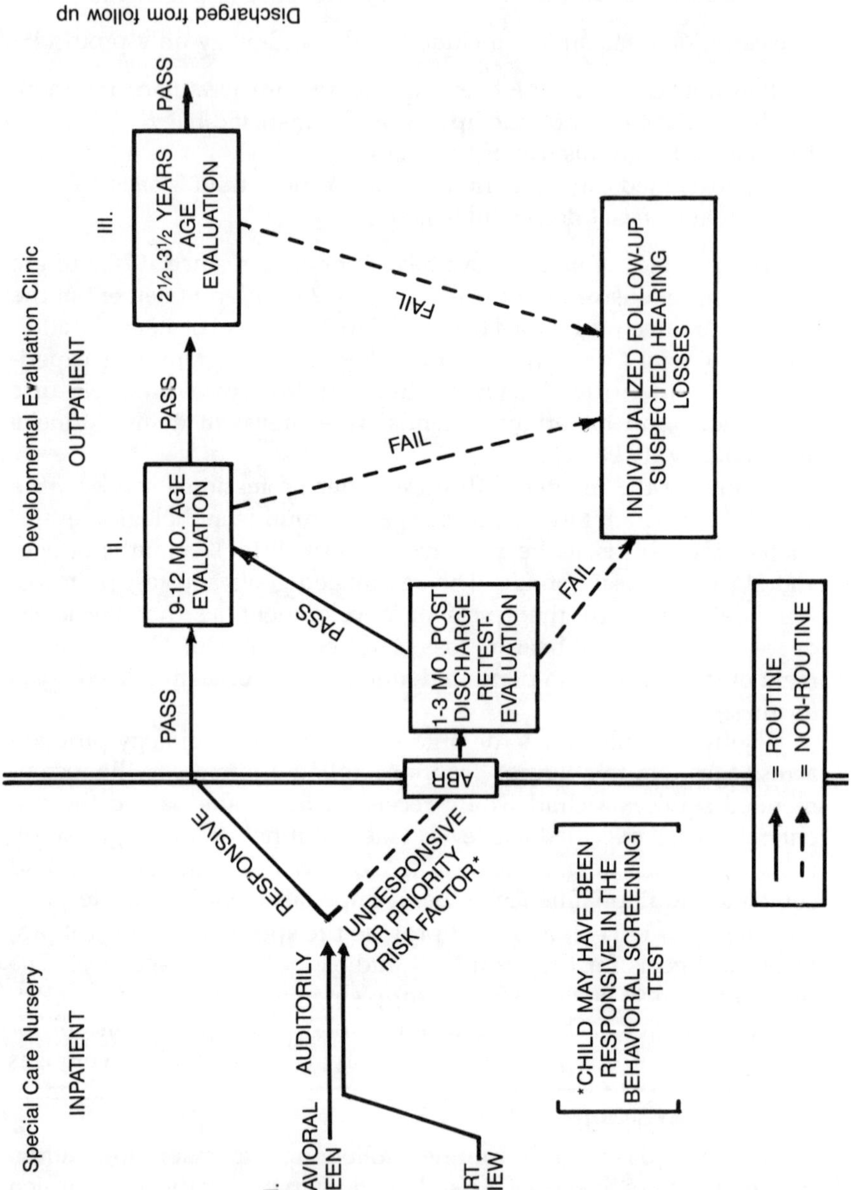

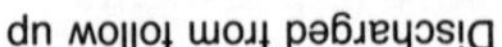

Figure 11-1. Screening and follow-up schedule.

TABLE 11–1.   Routine—Special Care Nursery

Audiological Protocol	Supplemental Goals
1. Medical chart review. 2. Behavioral auditory screening with retesting as necessary.	*Medical:* 1. Otoscopic examination of auditorily unresponsive infants may reveal undetected ear disease. 2. Visual examination of external ears to detect any subtle abnormalities that may warrant further evaluation.
Audiological Goals 1. Identify the auditorily unresponsive child (Qualitative). 2. Determine the presence of high-risk factors that warrant special follow-up recommendations.	*Developmental:* 1. Followup auditorily unresponsive infants to determine whether there are any significant problems in the group later cleared for hearing.

TABLE 11–2.   Routine—9 to 12 Months of Age

Audiological Protocol	Supplemental Goals
1. Sound-field testing with frequency-specific stimuli. 2. Behavioral observations of localization abilities. 3. Attempt to obtain some earphone measurement bilaterally. 4. Attempt to obtain tympanograms bilaterally.	*Medical:* 1. Identification of hearing loss may serve as an index of suspicion to explore the possibility of other problems. 2. Identify infants in need of otological follow-up.
Audiological Goals 1. Identify significant degrees of hearing loss that were previously undetected. 2. Rule out all degrees of bilateral hearing loss of more than a mild degree. 3. Rule out bilateral frequency-specific losses (primary speech range). 4. Try to detect any significant differences in sensitivity between ears.	*Developmental:* 1. Estimate level of auditory development to be included with other observations by team. 2. Observe infant's test performance: ability to condition, presence of perseverative behaviors, inconsistencies in performance. 3. Accumulate history and observational information on early speech and language development.

TABLE 11–3. Routine—2½ to 3½ Years of Age

Audiological Protocol	**Supplemental Goals**
1. Obtain complete threshold audiogram under earphones.	*Medical:*
2. Attempt to obtain complete impedance results.	1. Referral of newly identified cases of hearing loss.
3. Obtain some measure of speech discrimination under earphones, or in a quiet sound field.	2. Referral of cases warranting otological follow-up.
4. Measure speech discrimination in the sound field, in noise.	*Developmental:*
Audiological Goals	1. Referral to team for further testing if child's over-all test performance is of concern.
1. Clear the child for peripheral hearing loss.	2. Referral for speech and language evaluation if history or observations suggest concern or if a hearing loss is detected.
2. Identify unilateral, frequency-specific or mild degrees of loss.	3. Referral for additional testing if an auditory perceptual problem is suspected.
3. Detect gross speech discrimination deficits.	
4. Highlight possible gross auditory perceptual problems.	

only on the results of the actual auditory screening but also on the outcome of the chart review process. Infants with TORCH infections that could be associated with progressive hearing loss (rubella, syphilis, cytomegalovirus), those with a family history of hearing impairment, as well as those with significant visual problems are designated ''priority risk'' and are treated as though they were screening failures, being followed on a non-routine basis. For the nursery, non-routine follow-up includes a baseline ABR evaluation, performed as close as possible to the infant's discharge, with in-depth audiological follow-up 1 to 3 months post-discharge.

Using the nursery as an initial point to categorize routine from non-routine care permits planning and parent counseling prior to the infant's discharge. The utilization of routine follow-up also provides parents with the knowledge that their child will be evaluated again, regardless of the results of the initial screening. Infants who pass in the nursery, as well as those who fail, are reassessed at scheduled intervals not only to confirm the initial impression but also to add information about the auditory status of the developing child. Two full-time parent–infant educators work with parents whose infants are in the nursery or enrolled in DEC and remind the parent of services that their child will receive and the rationale for each service.

NICU infants are referred to the audiology program 1 to 2 weeks prior to their anticipated discharge from the nursery. The referrals are handled by the NICU discharge planning nurses, who refer only at-risk infants. Well babies with audiological risk factors are also referred to the program through the NICU discharge planning nurses as soon as their status is known. Most well babies are seen as inpatients, but because of their short hospital stay, some are seen 1 to 3 weeks post-discharge. Prior to being screened, all referred infants receive an independent chart review performed by the audiologist to ensure at-risk status, to record details of the medical history, and to record the DEC status (active or inactive). As a prerequisite to the screening, the infant must be off all life-support equipment and preferably off any ototoxic medications. Infants on apnea monitors and those receiving tube feedings are screened if they are otherwise healthy enough to be in an open crib. Occasionally, a baby who is still in an isolette requires a screening; in such instances, the baby is moved to an open crib for the duration of the screening to standardize the test and stimulus environment.

SCREENING METHOD

In 1977, when this program was established, the Joint Committee on Infant Hearing had issued its 1972 statement, which allowed for the assessment of at-risk infants only, and specified referral for "an in-depth audiological evaluation during the first two months of life." The Nova Scotia Conference on the Early Identification of Hearing Loss (Mencher, 1976) had resolved that, as a supplement to a high-risk register, an agency could use a behavioral test protocol and specified a model protocol. The other test method in use at the time was the prototype Crib-o-gram, and field studies with this unit were already in progress. Thus, if the audiology department was to conduct a hearing screening program in keeping with professional sanctions, there really was no choice of methods other than a behavioral screening. The decision to apply a behavioral screening was further justified, because all screenings were administered by experienced audiologists, usually with the assistance of a graduate student in audiology. Non-audiology personnel have not been involved in any portion of the program, other than the initial referral of infants. The test method for screening has always been considered an open-ended decision. If, at any time, program results suggest the need for a change, the method of testing in the nursery could be altered within the current program structure.

SCREENING PROTOCOL

The actual screenings are performed in a separate carpeted and furnished room in the nursery area. An infant can be screened up to a maximum of three times, and if he or she passes any of the subsequent screenings, he or she is considered to have passed.

State of the Infant at Testing

Every effort is made to control the infant's test state. A light sleep is desirable, but quiet alertness is also acceptable. Infants are usually removed from the bassinets and unwrapped so that body movement is most easily observed.

Stimuli

1. 3000 Hz warble tone stimulus is produced by a Zenith ZA 440 for 1 to 2 seconds. A maximum of six stimuli will be given for a single test session.
2. Narrowband noise with a center frequency of 500 or 3000 Hz is produced by an Amplaid Reactometer for 1 to 2 seconds.
3. The minimum interval between stimuli presentations is 15 seconds, but it is usually longer.
4. Initial stimuli intensities are 90 dB SPL. Subsequent stimuli are presented at 90 dB SPL again or increased to 100 dB SPL, dependent upon, respectively, the presence or absence of a response to the previous stimulus.

Response Scale

1. Acceptable responses for the 3000 Hz warble tone follow: **For sleeping infants**—(a) opening of the eyes; (b) stirring movement of the whole body, indicating an arousal from sleep; and (c) strong and immediate eye blinking followed by one of the first two responses. **For awake infants**—generalized body movement involving more than one limb and accompanied by eye movement and being clearly different from the baseline state. Responses are graded according to magnitude: 1 = no response observed; 2 = movement seen but doubtfully related to stimuli or obscured response; 3 = weak, but clearly a response; 4 = strong response; and 5 = paroxysmal response.
2. Responses to narrowband noise stimuli are not assigned a numerical rating for several reasons. First, this system of rating responses was suggested for warble tone stimuli by the Nova Scotia conference. Therefore, infants passing the criteria for warble tones receive a ''high-confidence'' pass. Second, behavioral

responses to narrowband noise stimuli are generally stronger and differ in type from those seen to warble tones. Thus, these responses are noted by appropriate descriptors, that is, arousing, startling, moro response, or crying, and are assigned a + or − symbol for tabulating purposes.

Pass Criteria

1. 3000 Hz warble tone stimulus—at least two responses of 3 or greater magnitude must be observed from one ear during the six allowable trials. In some questionable cases, the audiologist may make a clinical judgment to pass an infant who does not meet the specific guidelines. Examples of such cases would be infants who repeatably demonstrate a response pattern that is not one of the specified patterns, that is, a repeatable strong eye blink without eye opening in an asleep baby, post-stimulus vocalization, or a decrease in activity (quieting response) in an awake baby. If the infant is a clinical judgment pass, this is so recorded at the time of testing.

2. Narrowband noise stimuli—the baby must respond to each frequency (500 and 3000 Hz) during the two allowable trials on each side. If an infant responds only to noise-type stimuli, the best decision he or she can receive is a clinical judgment pass. Clinical judgment passes are considered as a lower confidence decision than an outright pass. This status does not change the infant's initial follow-up, because it is considered as passing versus failing. However, it is theoretically more likely that a child with a lesser degree of hearing loss, a frequency-specific loss, or a unilateral hearing loss could pass the screening under this clinical judgment "low confidence" pass. The accuracy of this initial decision will be judged at the time of the follow-up visits.

Follow-up ABR

ABR testing is completed on selected infants for whom immediate concerns regarding their auditory status cannot be resolved by behavioral testing. Included in this group are infants who have failed the nursery behavioral screening two to three times and infants with priority risk factors. In addition, infants who are being placed in foster or adoptive homes are also routinely seen for ABR testing upon the request of the managing physician. The infants are seen for ABR testing following the behavioral evaluation and as close to discharge as feasible.

The ABR test is conducted with the infants in a quiet natural sleep whenever possible. In very selected instances, mild sedation may be used to calm agitated infants. Tone pips or clicks are used as stimuli and are presented monaurally through handheld shielded earphones at a rate of 21.7 per second. The initial presentation level is 80 dB nHL. The intensity is then decreased in 20 dB steps until no repeatable response is observed or 40 dB nHL is reached. If a response is not present at 80 dB nHL, the stimulus level is raised to a maximum level of 90 dB nHL. The evaluation of the ABR includes the absence or presence of waveforms and absolute as well as interwave latency measures when possible. All responses are evaluated relative to the infant's known neurological and developmental status. A decision is then made as to the "normalcy" of the response for both hearing and neurological considerations. In all instances, the ABR is correlated to the behavioral results. In view of the confounding maturational factors, amplification is not recommended for the neonate based on the ABR results alone. In most instances, the infant is seen for priority follow-up in 1 to 3 months, at which time further testing and recommendations are completed.

REPORTING OF RESULTS

The outcome of the screening is recorded in the infant's medical chart under the daily progress note section. Infants who pass the screening receive the following stamped report:

Date: ______________________________

Audiology/High-Risk Hearing Screening: This infant was screened using a behavioral assessment of responses noted to a high-frequency (3000 Hz) warble tone of 80 and 90 dB HL intensity. Based on our observations, we consider this infant *cleared* at this time for a hearing loss of a severe degree bilaterally.

Given that this infant's at-risk status warranted screening, it is recommended that observational follow-up of auditory, speech, and language development be conducted by the pediatrician and that this child be referred for re-evaluation if concerns arise. Please notify the audiology department if this child is ever identified as being hearing impaired. (312) 908-8107 Northwestern University Hearing Services.

Clinical judgment passes—and failures—receive individually written hospital chart notes, because they are considered irregular and individualized decisions.

A copy of the chart information is sent to DEC or to the infant's private physician or both. For those infants who failed the behavioral screening and then received an ABR, a separate medical chart consultation report is written by the audiologist conducting the evaluation. A follow-up letter is written to DEC and to the physician when a hearing loss is confirmed with this combination of behavioral and

ABR techniques. Generally, all information regarding the child is routed through the team.

ADMINISTRATION AND COST CONSIDERATIONS

The nursery screening phase of the program takes 2 half-days to administer in an average week. The audiologist in charge of the program must also have sufficient scheduling flexibility to accommodate re-evaluations and tests of well babies. This program has been primarily administered by a single staff audiologist from 1977 to 1984. It is important that the audiologist testing the infants and working with the nursery personnel is familiar with the program so that it is routinely implemented and standardized.

The nursery screening is charged at the same rate as an outpatient children's evaluation. Currently, the charge per infant is $66, which is billed with the infant's hospital charges. As a comparison, this fee is less than the cost of one total and direct blood bilirubin level at this center. Payment for the screening is made to the hospital through private or public insurance carriers or through the parents. If a child was retested in the nursery, only one fee is assessed for all the behavioral testings. An ABR evaluation is a separate fee, once again being charged at the regular clinic rate for outpatients receiving this test. Probably the most important single factor in the success of this program is the fact that the first outpatient follow-up visit, usually at 9 to 12 months of age, is free if a baby was screened in the nursery. This "free re-evaluation" was established to eliminate fees from hindering the program's follow-up efforts. The accuracy of the nursery screening is best verified with a high return rate at 9 to 12 months for both screening passes and failures. The second routine follow-up visit at 2½ to 3½ years of age is billed at one half the usual children's appointment fee for outpatient visits. Every effort is made by the audiology department to provide evaluations to this population. This philosophy enhances the DEC team's effort on behalf of the audiology program. Although this program is not highly profitable, it was not established for that purpose. However, it is financially self-sufficient, and the current fee schedule seems workable.

FOLLOW-UP METHOD

The recommended audiological follow-up visits are initiated by DEC as a routine part of the care provided if a child is being followed by the team. It is estimated that 90 percent of the infants receiving audiological screenings become DEC cases, greatly simplifying follow-up efforts. For non-DEC cases, the pediatrician or the parent may initiate the referral for follow-up. Unfortunately, experience with referrals from sources other than DEC has been disappointing. Suffice it to say that a systematic referral system is ideal.

At the time of the DEC referral for the 9- to 12-month visit, the parents are given a letter from Audiology Services (Appendix 11-A). A second copy of this letter is placed in the child's file to alert the physician attending the developmental clinic to check whether the recommended audiological visit took place. If the parent did not keep the audiological follow-up appointment, DEC usually assists with rescheduling the child. The 3-month age range from 9 to 12 months for this appointment allows for evaluations of normally developing term babies earlier and premature or developmentally delayed babies later. In some instances, severe maturational delays warrant adjusting the re-evaluations in an individualized manner.

The testing of 2½ to 3½-year-old children has been less successful for a number of reasons. Many parents have dropped out of DEC by that age, especially those whose children are progressing normally. At this age, parents have numerous indications to subjectively assess a child's hearing. In addition, there is a fee for this visit. The audiological protocols for each of these ages are listed in Tables 11-2 and 11-3.

HABILITATION

The decision to establish a screening program must be accompanied by the responsibility for directing any necessary additional diagnostic or habilitative steps; a screening program in isolation is of limited value.

The amount of time spent in habilitation is directly related to the number of children identified as hearing impaired and the nature of any management plans. In a metropolitan area, there are multiple choices available for referral of hearing-impaired infants. The audiology program's goal has been to have any significantly hearing-impaired high-risk infants fitted with amplification and enrolled in programs as soon as possible, but, it is hoped, by 1 year of age. That sounds very lenient, but it has proved to be a difficult task in many cases. The Joint Committee on Infant Hearing, Position Statement (1982) recommends that habilitation begin by 6 months of age. Although theoretically this concept has been supported and viewed as ideal, over the past seven years, it has not been possible to meet this criterion. These infants are often at risk for more than hearing loss. Inherent in the choice to band with DEC and the other participating professionals was the decision to balance audiological management in proportion to any other problems the child may exhibit. Between medical complications, parental problems, and bureaucratic constrictions, the program audiologist's task is quite complex.

This center provides no direct outpatient therapy for hearingimpaired infants. Such services are available at the Evanston Campus of Northwestern University, as well as through other hospitals and public and private schools in the area. However, inpatients in need of habilitative care do receive services. In one instance, a chronically ill infant who was still hospitalized at 9 months of age was identified as hearing impaired. Intensive habilitation was initiated and provided on a daily basis during the remaining 6 months of his hospitalization.

The essential problem with habilitative management of cases in an NICU such as this is the broad base of the population served. Cases from a large metropolitan area plus several adjoining states make it necessary to constantly develop individual habilitative plans that best suit each infant. It is here that the parent–infant educators are of immeasurable assistance in evaluating programs, families, and infants with a perspective that is different from the audiologist's.

RESULTS OF THE NURSERY SCREENING

The yearly statistics and over-all totals of the years 1977–1984 are shown in Table 11–4. The number of infants tested per year has stabilized over the past 6 years and averages about 200 babies yearly. Although the initial failure rates were relatively high, 17.8 and 11.6 percent, they have decreased to more manageable levels, near 6 percent for the last 6 years. The decrease is thought to be related to a number of factors:

1. The use of the clinical judgment criterion for infants responsive to narrowband noise has a direct implication on the failure rate. Essentially, this category has reduced the number of failures by allowing a lower confidence pass.
2. Discharge planning nurses were implemented in the nursery in 1979. They were able to accurately inform the audiology department of the anticipated discharge dates for the infants; this permitted testing of infants closer to discharge when the infants were larger and healthier.
3. The same audiologists were involved in the program for 4 to 8 years. Consistency in making behavioral judgments in addition to ongoing experience with this population contributed to a stabilization of failure rates.

TABLE 11–4. Results of the Nursery Screening

	1977	1978	1979	1980	1981	1982	1983	1984	Totals
Tested	146	147	202	179	177	210	202	203	1466
High-Confidence Pass	120	130	189	159	139	177	157	157	1228
Clinical Judgment, Lower Confidence Pass	*	*	*	8	30	23	42	38	141
Failed	26	17	13	12	8	10	3	8	97
(%)	(17.8)	(11.6)	(6.4)	(6.7)	(4.5)	(4.8)	(1.5)	(4.0)	(6.6)
Hearing Impaired	2	3	4	4	3	4	1	4	25†
Incidence	1:73	1:49	1:50	1:45	1:44	1:50	1:202	1:51	1:59

* Clinical judgment passes were instituted in 1980.

† Two of these children passed the screening with mild hearing losses but were identified at follow-up testing.

The overall average incidence of hearing loss has been 1 in 59, whereas individual years have ranged from 1 in 44 in 1981 to 1 in 202 in 1983. This figure for 1983 is clearly discrepant from the other yearly incidence figures. During this year, a number of very ill infants received clinical judgment passes on the nursery screening but died prior to receiving follow-up services. It is speculated that due to a high mortality rate in this group, morbidity, that is, hearing loss, was not fully identified. The Joint Committee's 1982 statement suggests an incidence figure of 2½ to 5 percent, or 1 in 40 to 1 in 20, for moderate to profound hearing loss to be used as a target figure in planning. The majority of this screening program's incidence figures are close to the 1:40 figure, and the follow-up program adds further strength to the audiological identification efforts.

The false-negative rate (infants who passed the screening and were later found to be hearing impaired) was 12.5 percent, or 2 of 25 infants. Both of these infants had hearing losses too mild to be detected in the behavioral screening procedure. Although it is desirable to decrease this number even further, the comprehensive follow-up plan for this program, coupled with a good return for services, is an important consideration. These two children were still quite young when identified as mildly hearing impaired. Without a systematic program, such cases would probably not be identified until symptoms developed or the child reached preschool or school age.

ABR testing was incorporated into the program in 1980 as a supplement, not a substitute for the behavioral protocol. Since incorporating this test procedure, hearing losses have been confirmed at significantly earlier ages, usually prior to the infant's discharge from the hospital, and the degree of hearing loss has been delineated.

Although having these test results is diagnostically favorable, early diagnosis has not reliably led to the anticipated earlier habilitation of these infants. In a practical sense, it seems that, currently, the greater professional challenge is not the identification of hearing loss, but securing the remediation of the hearing-impaired high-risk child at an age when the child's potential can be maximized.

SUMMARY

The undertaking of a screening program is a considerable professional responsibility, the success of which is dependent upon numerous variables. Even the most concerned audiologist can do little through a singular effort with this population. This program could not have continued if the sponsoring hospital was not vested in the follow-up of these children. Retrospectively, the planning of the program, which took almost a year, is still considered to be the best investment, and individuals involved in initiating new programs are urged to carefully weigh all aspects of program management prior to beginning to screen infants. The task of identification and habilitation is confounded by the nature of the infants, the multidisciplinary aspects of their care, and the diversity and complexity of the family structures represented. The provision of identification and follow-up services to high-risk infants is clearly an area in which only the most professional audiological efforts should be directed.

ACKNOWLEDGMENT

The author wishes to recognize the sizable contribution of her colleague and co-worker in this program for a number of years, as she contributed to the ultimate organization of this project:
Karen M. Gollegly, M.A.
Dartmouth-Hitchcock Medical Center
Hanover, NH 03755

REFERENCES

Joint Committee on Infant Hearing Screening, Supplemental statement (1974). *ASHA, 16*(3), 160.
Joint Committee on Infant Hearing, Position statement (1982). *ASHA, 24*(12), 1017–1018.
Mencher, G. T. (Ed.) (1976). *Early identification of hearing loss.* Basel: S. Karger.
Moneka, W. J., and Gollegly, K. M. (1983, November). *The design and results of a high-risk hearing screening program.* Paper presented at the annual convention of the American Auditory Society, Cincinnati, OH.

Appendix **11–A**

Letter Sent to Parents of 9- to 12-Month-Old Children

YOUR CHILD NEEDS FOLLOW-UP HEARING TESTING

Dear Parent:

You may remember that your baby had a hearing test before leaving the Special Care Nursery. That testing was performed because many of the problems that require intensive medical care in the newborn period are also known to be associated with a slightly increased risk of hearing loss. The nursery screening of a baby's hearing is only the first step in hearing loss detection. Very young babies can only be checked reliably for severe degrees of hearing loss, but, as with any problem affecting a baby, early identification and treatment or therapy are the best keys in safeguarding the child's development.

At this time, we want to let you know that the Hearing Clinic offers a *free follow-up visit* for babies seen in the nursery. Your baby should be seen for this one-hour visit when he or she is between 9 and 12 months of age. Testing children of this age allows us to find milder degrees of hearing loss that would not have been detectable in the nursery screening and may not be obvious in the child's actions or developmental progress. Good hearing in infancy and childhood is essential for a child to talk and learn normally. *Even a mild hearing loss can affect a baby's development in this critical period.*

Please call our Clinic at 908-8107 to request an *at-risk follow-up appointment* for your child. This testing will be done by examiners experienced in testing young children, and they will have your baby's past hearing screening records available for reference. (If you baby *was not* seen in the hospital for a hearing screening or was seen before July 11, 1978, a modest charge will be assigned for this testing.)

Sincerely,

Hearing Services

Chapter **12**
MODEL PROGRAM IV

A High-Risk Register, Crib-o-gram, and Auditory Brainstem Response

**The Reading Hospital and Medical Center
Reading, Pennsylvania**

Elca T. Swigart

The Reading Hospital and Medical Center is a 654-bed community hospital where more than 2,000 live births take place each year. Although the hospital contains a Level II intensive care nursery, neonates requiring more acute care are transferred to nearby facilities that house Level III intensive care units.

Neonatal hearing screening was initiated at this hospital in November 1981. Minor revisions took place in 1982, and the current program has been in operation since that time.

PROGRAM DEVELOPMENT

The first step in Reading Hospital's program was investigation by the audiologist to determine the feasibility of a neonatal hearing screening program with respect to time, cost, and personnel constraints at this hospital. Although auditory brainstem response (ABR) equipment was available, the professional time and cost of test administration to screen all infants at risk seemed prohibitive. Therefore, an alternate screening method was sought. From published reports through 1980, the Crib-o-gram procedure appeared to have promise. It was thought that immediate ABR screening for the limited number of Crib-o-gram referrals would be possible and would reduce the number of unnecessary referrals for extended follow-up.

Thus, a protocol that included a high-risk register, Crib-o-gram, and ABR screening was developed.

Prior to 1981, the Joint Committee on Infant Hearing had recommended five high-risk factors. Several investigators (Cone, 1980; Feinmesser and Tell, 1974; and Simmons, McFarland and Jones, 1980) had also been analyzing additional risk factors. Since the Crib-o-gram was chosen as a screening technique, special consideration was given to those high-risk factors studied by Simmons and reported in various studies with Crib-o-gram screening. Thus, in addition to the five factors suggested by the 1972 Joint Committee on Infant Hearing, the high-risk register at this hospital included six additional factors (Table 12–1).

Difficulties encountered during the first year of screening included equipment failure for both ABR and Crib-o-gram. After all systems appeared to be working smoothly, data analysis of the high-risk factors and screening results indicated that a much larger percent of infants was considered at risk (30 percent) than was expected. In previous reports of hearing screening in the general newborn population, Mencher (1974) and Northern and Downs (1978) had found only 6 to 7 percent at risk. Item analysis of the high-risk factors at this hospital indicated an unusually high proportion of risk for "family history of hearing loss," placement in an "intensive care nursery," and "difficult delivery" items. The high percent of neonates with family history of hearing loss was not unexpected, because nurses were originally instructed to screen all neonates with a relative reported to have any kind of hearing loss that occurred before the age of 5 years if the loss still existed in the relative. Regarding the "intensive care" category, further investigation revealed that most of the graduates of that unit were found to have no other risk factors. The high risk for neonates in the intensive care nursery previously reported in the literature apparently applied to Level III nurseries only. Finally, the attending physicians interpreted "difficult delivery" in a very liberal manner, and, again, most neonates identified with difficult delivery had no other risk criteria. Based on this information, a more restrictive high-risk register was considered. At approximately the same time, the 1982 Joint Committee on Infant Hearing suggested a seven-item register that closely resembled the limited register under consideration. The risk factors recommended by the Joint Committee and now in use at this hospital are listed in Table 12–1.

SCREENING PROTOCOL

Table 12–2 outlines the hearing screening protocol from birth through 1 year of age. As illustrated in the outline, the procedure

Table 12–1.   High–Risk Registers Used Initially (left) and Currently (right)

*Family history of childhood hearing impairments	†Family history of childhood hearing impairments
*Congenital perinatal infection	†Congenital perinatal infection
Intensive care nursery	†Defects of ear, nose, or throat
*Defects of ear, nose, or throat	†Low birthweight
*Low birthweight less than 1500 gm	†High bilirubin level
*Bilirubin level greater than 20 mg	†Neonatal meningitis
Neonatal sepsis	†Severe asphyxia
Neonatal meningitis	Other _________________
Difficult delivery	
Respiratory distress	
Low Apgar score	

*Recommended by Joint Committee on Infant Hearing in 1972.

†Recommended by Joint Committee on Infant hearing in 1982.

Table 12–2.   Flow Chart for Neonatal Hearing Screening at The Reading Hospital and Medical Center

In-Hospital

Mother's interview—mother given pamphlet concerning baby's hearing

High-risk register

   Pass—no further follow-up
   Fail—screen with Crib-o-gram

Crib-o-gram

   Pass—no further follow-up until 1-year questionnaire

   Fail—screen with ABR

ABR Screening (results to pediatrician)

   Pass—No further follow-up until 1-year questionnaire

   Fail—ABR at 3 months

After Release From Hospital

Threshold ABR at 3 months of age (results to pediatrician)

   Pass—no further follow-up until 1-year questionnaire

   Fail—complete audiological evaluation at 7 months

Complete audiological evaluation at 7 months (results to pediatrician)

   Pass—no further follow-up until 1-year questionnaire

   Fail—A. If still *suspect* for *mild hearing* loss, recommend continued audiological and possibly medical surveillance.

      B. If diagnostic tests suggest *moderate* to *profound hearing loss*, appropriate procedures should be followed for habilitation (medical clearance for amplification, hearing aid evaluation and fitting, and referral to the local Preschool Hearing-Impaired Program).

Follow-up questionnaire at 1 year for all babies at risk

includes the determination of risk, the screening, the audiological follow-up testing for diagnosis, and initial habilitative procedures.

High-Risk Register

Included in every newborn baby's chart is a neonatal hearing screening form (Appendix 12–A). This form contains items on the high-risk register, the mother's questionnaire, and spaces for recording Crib-o-gram and ABR screening results. The form is duplicated on a second sheet of pressure sensitive paper. When completed, the original stays in the baby's chart, and the copy is sent to the Speech and Hearing Center, where the coordinator of the screening is based.

All mothers are interviewed by a nurse (see mother's questionnaire in Appendix 12–A) and are given a pamphlet concerning the baby's hearing (Appendix 12–B). If the results of the interview suggest a risk for hearing loss, a check is placed on the high-risk register (Appendix 12–A). The baby's chart is also reviewed by the nurse for other risk criteria. The nurses are given detailed instructions concerning the mothers' interviews and the completion of the screening forms through instructional sessions and an instructional pamphlet (Appendix 12–C). The nursing staff reports that the completion of the high-risk register may take from 2 to 8 minutes depending on the complication of the case or the explanations needed to encourage the mother to respond correctly.

Crib-o-gram Screening

If the baby is considered at risk for hearing by one or more criteria, he or she is screened with the Crib-o-gram. The Crib-o-gram screening is a nursing procedure supervised by the audiologist and is done in the nursery where the baby is located. The screening is done one day prior to the baby's release from the hospital. This time frame permits immediate ABR screening if the baby does not pass the Crib-o-gram screening.

If the baby does not pass Crib-o-gram screening, the attending pediatrician is alerted by the nurses that further auditory screening is recommended. The pediatrician may also gain this information from the neonatal hearing screening form kept in the baby's hospital chart. The nurses also notify the Speech and Hearing Center by phone when ABR screening has been requested.

Time to administer the Crib-o-gram screening includes approximately 2 to 3 minutes to set up and 2 to 3 minutes to take down and record the response. The actual testing time of the Crib-o-gram procedure ranges from 15 minutes to one-half hour.

Auditory Brainstem Response Screening

ABR screening is administered by a staff audiologist either in the nursery or in the mother's room, whichever provides the more quiet environment after the baby has been fed and is asleep. Pediatric Grass electrodes are placed at the vertex and mastoid areas with Grass CE 2 electrode cream and Micropure Hypoallergenic tape after preparation with Omni Prep paste. Click stimuli from a Nicolet CA-1000 unit are presented at 40 dB (re: normal adult threshold) in rarefaction phase through TDH-39 earphones at the rate of 13 per second. Two tracings of 2000 sweeps are obtained for each ear. If the latency of Wave V falls within expected limits as indicated by normative data from healthy, full-term neonates at this hospital, the baby passes the screening. ABR screening, which includes acquisition of parental permission, sterilization of equipment, testing, and reporting results to parent, takes approximately 30 minutes.

Screening results are noted in the hospital chart under the previous terminology, Brainstem Evoked Response Audiometry. If the baby passes the ABR screening, a letter is sent to the pediatrician indicating that the baby passed the second screening, and no further formal audiological follow-up is requested (Appendix 12–D). However, the parents and pediatricians are encouraged to observe the baby's responses to auditory stimuli for the new few months.

If the baby does not pass the ABR screening, a letter is sent to the pediatrician indicating the need for further testing to clarify hearing sensitivity (Appendix 12–E), and the baby's name is placed on a 3-month recall file in the Speech and Hearing Center. The pediatrician may at any time request an otological or a neurological examination or both.

In the event that the baby and the mother are released from the hospital over a weekend, and there has been no ABR screening following a Crib-o-gram referral, the baby is recalled in 3 months for ABR testing. A letter is sent to the pediatrician indicating the need for recall (Appendix 12–F).

Auditory Brainstem Response Testing at Three Months

The parents are sent a letter indicating the appointment time and date for the 3-month test (Appendix 12–G), which involves ABR threshold assessment. The patient preparation is the same as that described for the screening, and testing is administered in a quiet audiology office.

If the child passes the 3-month ABR retest, a letter is sent to the pediatrician indicating that hearing loss is not suspected (Appendix

12–H) and no further audiological follow-up is requested. Because hearing loss can occur in a high-risk population after birth, the parents and pediatricians are advised to observe the child's responses to auditory stimuli for the next few months.

If, however, the child does not pass the 3-month ABR test, a letter is sent to the pediatrician indicating the need for a complete audiological evaluation at 7 months of age (Appendix 12–I), and the child is placed in the 7-month recall file in the Speech and Hearing Center.

Complete Audiological Evaluation at Seven Months

At the appropriate time, a letter to the parents (Appendix 12–G) indicates an appointment date and time for a hearing test.

A complete audiological evaluation at 7 months of age includes behavioral observation audiometry, ABR threshold testing, and impedance audiometry, including tympanometry and assessment of stapedius reflexes. If the parents desire to have the testing done elsewhere, it is requested that a copy of the results be sent to the Speech and Hearing Center to complete the follow-up program.

If the child passes the 7-month complete audiological evaluation, a letter is sent to the pediatrician indicating that the child passed the hearing testing and no further audiological follow-up is requested (Appendix 12–J). However, the parents and pediatrician are encouraged to observe the child's responses to auditory stimuli for the next few months.

If the child's responses at 7 months suggest the possibility of a mild hearing loss, a letter is sent to the pediatrician indicating that the child should be followed audiologically until a more definite picture of the hearing sensitivity is obtained (Appendix 12–K). An otological evaluation is suggested to the pediatrician if it has not previously been obtained.

If the 7-month complete audiological evaluation suggests a moderate to severe hearing loss, a letter is sent to the pediatrician indicating that appropriate measures will be taken for habilitation (Appendix 12–L). This includes medical clearance for amplification (Appendix 12–M), hearing aid fitting, and referral to the area preschool hearing-impaired program. If the parents are doubtful concerning the existence of a significant hearing loss or are hesitant concerning the fitting of a hearing aid at this time, they are encouraged to seek a second opinion.

Questionnaire at One Year

At 1 year of age, follow-up letters (Appendix 12–N) and questionnaires (Appendix 12–O) are sent to the parents of all high-risk infants, whether or not the babies failed any screening tests. Because hearing impairments may occur in a high-risk population after birth, the purpose of this questionnaire is to alert the parents to any hearing difficulties, encourage them to discuss the matter with the child's pediatrician, and let them know that the child's hearing can be tested if there is any question concerning the child's hearing abilities.

ADMINISTRATIVE CONSIDERATIONS

After detailed planning and a year of modifications, the screening program is currently carried out with approximately 5 percent of the audiologist's time allocated to the screening program. This includes supervision of the high-risk register and Crib-o-gram screening, administration of ABR screening, and follow-up diagnostic testing for the first 7 months of life of each child with a suspected hearing loss. In addition, the coordinator collects and tabulates all data. To achieve this minimal time requirement, the audiologist's time is somewhat flexible to permit the administration of ABR screening before each child leaves the hospital. In addition, data collection is routinely followed by periodic tabulation.

A minimum of clerical time is required, because letters and reports are already prepared. An additional expense of printing information pamphlets and the pressure sensitive forms for recording high-risk or screening information has been greatly reduced by in-house printing and costs only a few cents per child.

There is a charge of $6 per Crib-o-gram screening. An ABR screening is one half the fee of a complete ABR evaluation. These are billed with the infant's hospital charges. Payment is made through insurance carriers or the parents. Payment for follow-up testing is made through insurance carriers or parents or application may be made to the State Department of Health for financial assistance.

RESULTS

From the initiation of the screening program in 1981 through the first few months of 1985, 7,354 live births occurred at Reading Hospital and Medical Center. Four infants with confirmed hearing losses greater than 40 dB HL have been identified: two with bilateral profound sensorineural losses, one with a moderate unilateral sensorineural loss, and one with a moderate bilateral conductive loss.

Figure 12–1 summarizes the screening since January, 1983, when the revised high-risk register was initiated. Of the total births, 372 (8 percent) were considered at risk. Crib-o-gram screening was adminis-

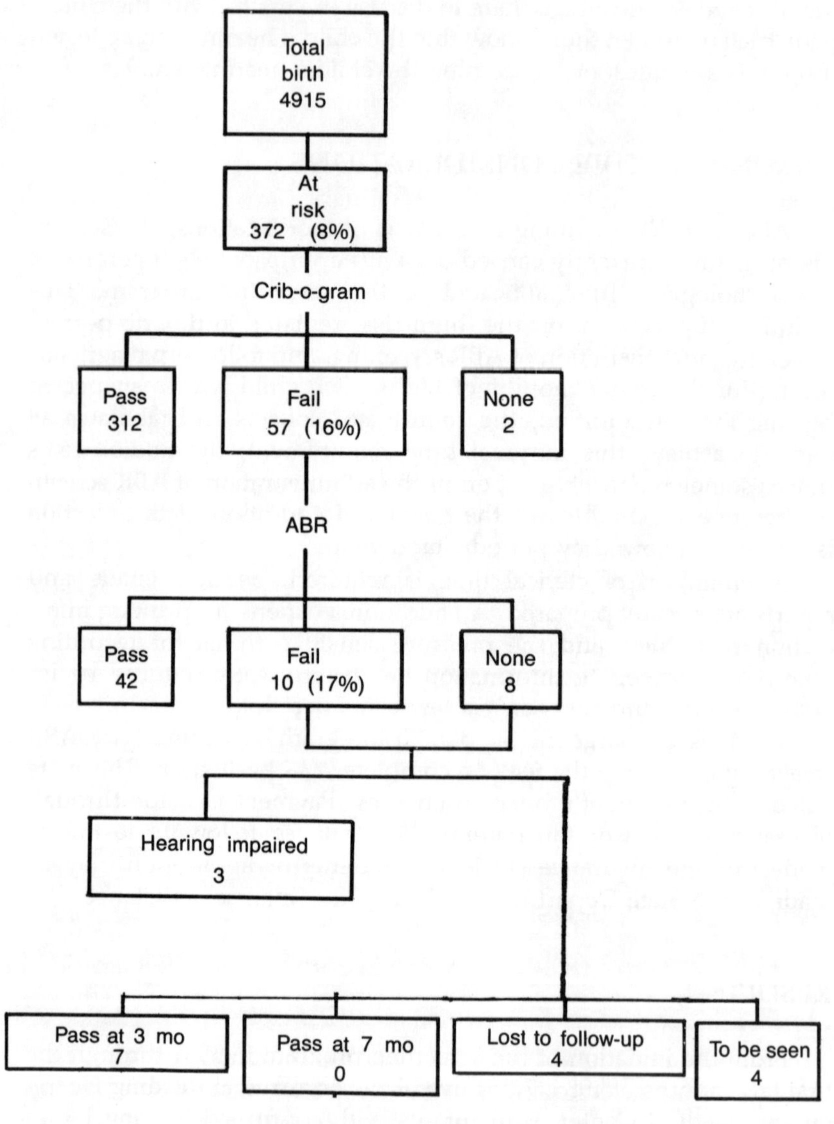

Figure 12–1. Summary of screening data from January, 1983, through March, 1985.

tered for all except two infants whose parents refused to give permission for the testing. Fifty-seven infants (16 percent of those at risk) failed the Crib-o-gram screening. Of the 57 who failed the Crib-o-gram screening, 10 (17 percent) also failed immediate ABR screening. Of the 18 infants who either failed immediate ABR screening or were not screened with ABR, 7 passed at the 3-month retest, 4 were lost to follow-up, 3 were hearing impaired and required audiological or medical management, and 4 are still to be evaluated.

The first column in Table 12–3 illustrates the percent of infants at risk for each of the risk categories. Only three infants were identified at risk by multiple factors. Although the percent at risk for family history is quite large, the high numbers were not unexpected, because nurses were originally instructed to screen any infant with a family history of early onset of hearing loss reported by the mother. If family members with reported hearing loss had been purged to exclude relatives other than siblings, parents, grandparents, aunts, uncles, and cousins and to exclude hearing loss as a result of trauma or disease at an early age or hearing loss possibly caused by a condition of pregnancy, the number of infants with reported family history would have been greatly reduced. Likewise, if mothers with congenital perinatal infection has been purged to exclude reports of rash in the second and third trimesters of pregnancy when the chance of developing congenital defects is small, the number in that category would have been significantly reduced. Finally, if all screenings upon parental request were excluded from the "other" category, the number of infants remaining would have been extremely small. By purging the data in the three categories just mentioned, the total neonatal population at risk is reduced from 8 percent to 5 percent.

The percent of Crib-o-gram failure was calculated for each risk category (the second column in Table 12–3). Because of the small number of infants in some of the categories, the data must be interpreted with caution.

The averages of the Crib-o-gram passing and failing scores were tabulated for each category. Because the cut-off for passing was 50, one might expect an average pass score of approximately 75. Under the Crib-o-gram "pass" column in Table 12–3, note that the average score ranged from 61 to 78. Under the "fail" column, note that the scores were similar among all categories and were just below the 50 cut-off for passing. All four infants with confirmed hearing loss registered Crib-o-gram scores ranging from 40 to 48.

Questionnaires were mailed to parents of all infants at risk, whether or not the infants passed the original screening. Four percent of the parents could not be reached because of changes of address. Sixty-three percent of the questionnaires were returned. Although the primary purpose of the questionnaire was to alert par-

Table 12–3. Analysis of Screening Data

	Percent of Total Infants at Risk	Percent of Crib-o-gram Failure	Average Crib-o-gram Score:	
			Pass	*Fail*
Family history of childhood hearing impairments	62	15	78	42
Congenital perinatal infection	12	19	80	43
Defects of ear, nose and throat	2	23	72	45
Low birthweight	3	23	61	47
High bilirubin level	0.3	—	71	—
Neonatal meningitis	0.3	—	77	—
Severe asphyxia	5	24	78	43
Other	16	14	75	40

ents to any possible progressive hearing loss, it was interesting to note that more than half of those responding (53 percent) indicated that the child had already experienced one or more ear infections in the first year.

SUMMARY

Although a higher percentage of infants with hearing loss is reportedly found in the intensive care nursery than in the general well-baby nursery, we cannot overlook the identification of hearing-impaired newborns who are otherwise healthy, normal-appearing babies. This screening program was designed to use available equipment and personnel to efficiently screen newborns in a community hospital that contained a well-baby nursery and a Level II intensive care nursery.

The success of the program has been dependent upon many elements. Perhaps the most outstanding factors were detailed planning for all aspects of the program from the initial screen through habilitative efforts, the dedication of the nursing staff, and the continued support of pediatricians.

In addition to identifying hearing-impaired neonates, thus permitting early habilitative efforts, the screening program has also provided an avenue to promote professional and lay awareness of hearing, hearing loss, and the importance of early identification of those who have hearing problems.

REFERENCES

Cone, B. (1980). Auditory evoked potentials for pediatric evaluations. *Audiology and Hearing Education, 6,* 7–11.

Feinmesser, M., and Tell, L. (1974). Evaluation of methods for detecting hearing impairment in infancy and early childhood. In G. T. Mencher (Ed.), *Early identification of hearing loss* (pp. 102–113). Basel: S. Karger.

Mencher, G. (1974). Infant hearing screening: The state of the art. *Maico Audiological Library Series, 12,* Report 7.

Northern, J., and Downs, M. (1978). *Hearing in children* (2nd ed.; p. 206). Baltimore: Williams and Wilkins.

Simmons, F., McFarland, W., and Jones, F. (1979). An automated hearing screening technique for newborns. *Acta Otolaryngology, 87,* 1–8.

Appendix **12–A**

Neonatal Hearing Screening Report Form

THE READING HOSPITAL AND MEDICAL CENTER

NEONATAL HEARING SCREENING

HIGH RISK REGISTER

A 1. Family history of (hereditary) childhood hearing   No___ Yes___
impairments
(See Mother's Questionnaire)

B 2. Congenital perinatal infection (eg. cytomegalo-   No___ Yes___
virus, rubella, herpes, toxoplasmosis, syphilis)
(See Mother's Questionnaire and Prenatal History)

C 4. Defects of the ear, nose or throat, malformed, low- No___ Yes___
set or absent pinnae; cleft lip or palate (including
submucous cleft); any residual abnormality of the
otorhinolaryngeal system
(See Labor and Delivery Summary and Initial
Newborn Profile)

D 5. Birthweight less than 1,500 grams   No___ Yes___
(See Labor & Delivery Summary)

E 6. Bilirubin level greater than 20 mg per 100 ml serum No___ Yes___
(See Lab Studies)

F 8. Neonatal Meningitis   No___ Yes___
(See Initial Newborn Profile)

G12. Severe Asphyxia - fail to initiate spontaneous   No___ Yes___
respiration by ten minutes, or hypotonia persisting
to two hours of age, or Apgar less than 4.
(See Labor & Delivery Summary)

H13. Other _________________________________   No___ Yes___

If there is a check in the "Yes" column, a Crib-O-Gram should be obtained.

Infant's
Name last______________________   first______________________

CRIB - O - GRAM
SCREENING

__________ **Pass**

__________ **Refer**

Cursor Number________________

Date________________ Tester________

If there is a check by "Refer", Brainstem Evoked
Response Audiometry should be requested.

Brainstem Evoked Response Audiometry

Date____________ Pass______

Retest___

Pediatrician's name:

____

MOTHER'S QUESTIONNAIRE

1 Do you know any of the baby's relatives who now have a hearing loss which started before the age of five?   Yes__________ No__________

   A. If **no**, proceed to question #2.

   B. If **yes**, ask the following:

     (a) Who were they? (relation to baby)

       1.__________ 2.__________ 3.__________

     (b) Do you know what caused the loss? Yes__________ No__________

       1.__________ 2.__________ 3.__________

     (c) What makes you think the onset of the hearing loss was before age five?

       1.__________ 2.__________ 3.__________

     (d) Did he/she wear a hearing aid before age five?

       1.__________ 2.__________ 3.__________

     (e) Did he/she attend a special school for the deaf?

       1.__________ 2.__________ 3.__________

     (f) Did he/she have a speech problem?

       1.__________ 2.__________ 3.__________

2. During your pregnancy, did you have Three-day Measles, German Measles, Rubella, or a rash with a fever?

   Yes__________ No__________

   WHEN: 1st 3 mo.__________ Middle 3 mo.__________ Last 3 mo.__________

3. During your pregnancy, were you around anyone who had Three-day Measles, German Measles, Rubella, or a rash with fever?

   Yes__________ No__________

   WHEN: 1st 3 mo.__________ Middle 3 mo.__________ Last 3 mo.__________

4. Do you have any reason to be concerned about your baby's hearing?

   Yes__________ No__________

   If yes, why __________________________________

5 What pediatrician or clinic will be caring for your baby when he/she leaves the hospital?__________________________________

Name

____

Location

____

Interviewer

(Revised January, 1983)

HEARING SCREENING

NEWBORN RECORD COPY

RH 2516

Appendix 12–B

Contents of Pamphlet Concerning Hearing Given to All Mothers

The content of this pamphlet was compiled by the Audiology Section of the University of Colorado Medical Center, in cooperation with the Listen Foundation, headquartered at Porter Memorial Hospital, in 1976. Minor changes were made by the Speech and Hearing Center of The Reading Hospital and Medical Center in 1981.

SPEECH AND HEARING CENTER
THE READING HOSPITAL AND MEDICAL CENTER
READING, PA   19603
(215)   378-6694

CAN YOUR BABY HEAR?

information for parents

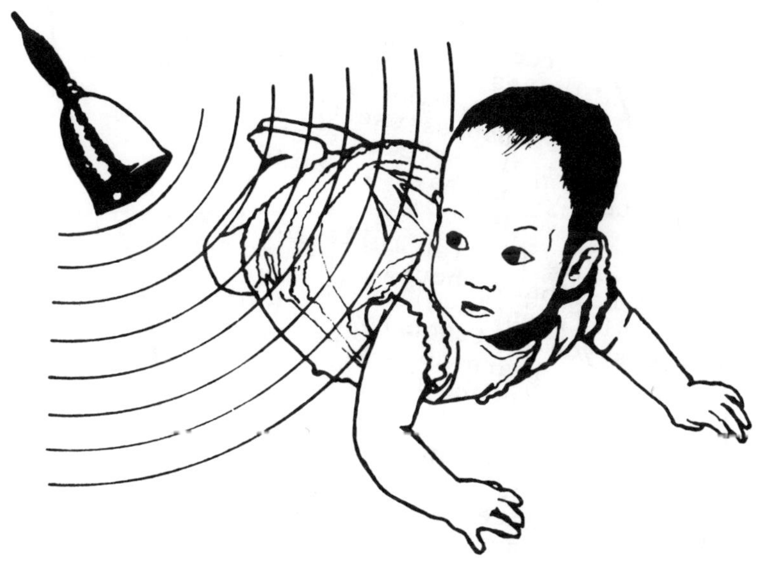

**The Speech and Hearing Center
The Reading Hospital
and Medical Center**

Dear Parents,

Your baby's ability to hear is very important for it helps determine his future social and physical development, especially his power of speech. If a hearing loss is found early, there are many things that can be done to help. But first this loss must be detected.

Mothers and fathers play a crucial role in finding hearing losses in young babies. Parents are also important in helping their babies use their hearing and learn speech, whether or not the babies have a hearing loss.

This booklet tells you how a normal baby should react to sound at different age levels. It also gives you hints on how to help your baby learn to use his hearing and speaking abilities.

If you have any questions, ask your doctor. The Speech and Hearing Center at The Reading Hospital and Medical Center will be here to help you if we're needed.

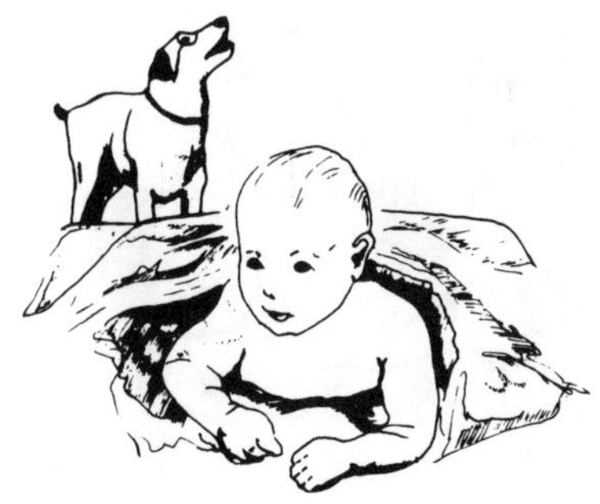

By <u>four months</u>, your baby should:

1. Stir or awaken when he is sleeping
    quietly and someone talks or makes
    a loud noise. (He doesn't always
    have to do this, but you should be
    able to notice it occasionally.)

2. Sometimes start or jump when there
    is a very loud sound, like a cough
    or a dog bark or a dish falling to
    the floor.

If your baby never does these things, or
if you have seen him do them only once,

        TELL THE BABY'S
        DOCTOR ABOUT IT.

What you should be doing:

1. Whenever he makes sounds, try to
    imitate them. When talking to him,
    use a pleasant voice.
2. Hold him close to you often, rocking
    or singing to him. Talk quietly to
    him.
3. Talk to him while you work around
    the house. "Hello, Johnny." Use
    his name.

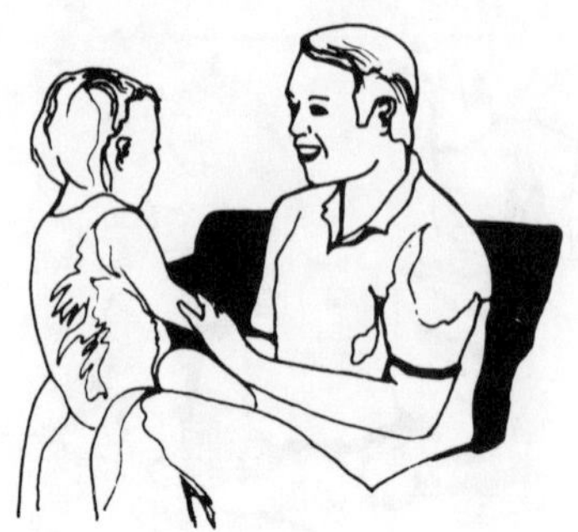

By <u>seven months</u>, your baby should:

1. Turn her head toward a sound or when
    her name is called when she cannot
    see you.
2. Stir or awaken when she is sleeping
    quietly and someone talks or makes
    a loud sound.
3. Sometimes start or jump when there
    is a very loud sound.

If your baby never does these things, or
if you have only seen her do them once,

        TELL THE BABY'S
        DOCTOR ABOUT IT.

What you should be doing:

1. Keep on imitating her sounds and
    then talk to her a lot.
2. Hold her close to you often, singing
    or talking to her.
3. Talk to her about her toys and play
    baby games with her ("Pat-a-cake,"
    "Up-you-go," "Peek-a-boo").

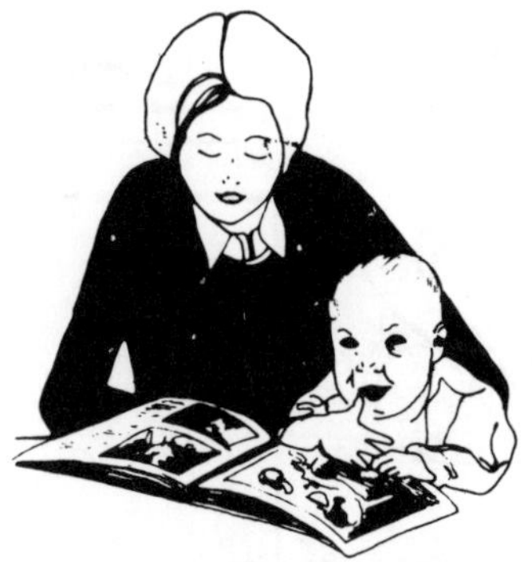

By <u>nine months</u>, your baby should:

1. Directly find a sound made at his side, or turn his head when you call him from behind.
2. Stir or awaken when he is sleeping quietly and someone talks or makes a loud sound.
3. Sometimes jump or start when there is a very loud sound.

If your baby never does these things, or if you have only seen him do them once,

TELL THE BABY'S
DOCTOR ABOUT IT.

What you should be doing:

1. Make simple speech sounds to see if he will imitate you ("buh-buh," "gah-gah," "ooh-ooh").
2. Pay some attention to him if he says "Mama," or "Dada."
3. Keep on talking to him about every-thing he plays with and about things in the house. Play singing games with him.
4. Show him pictures in books, and talk about them.

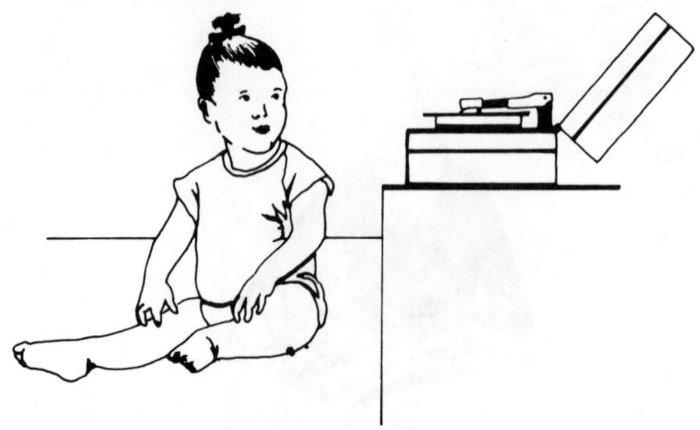

By <u>twelve months</u>, your baby should:

1. Turn her head in any direction and
    find an interesting sound or the
    person speaking.
2. Begin to repeat some of the sounds
    you make.
3. Stir or awaken when she is sleeping
    quietly and someone talks or makes
    a loud sound.

If your baby never does these things, or
if you have seen her do them only once,

TELL THE BABY'S
DOCTOR ABOUT IT.

What you should be doing:

1. Show her the parts of her body, "Here's
    the baby's nose," "here's the baby's
    ears," and put her hand to them.
2. Show her simple picture books, telling
    her to turn the pages. Talk about
    each picture.
3. Play "where's Daddy" (or "Mama") and
    point to Daddy (or Mama). Also,
    "where's the doggy" (or other toy) and
    point to it. Explain sounds - "What
    does the doggy say?" "Bow-Wow."

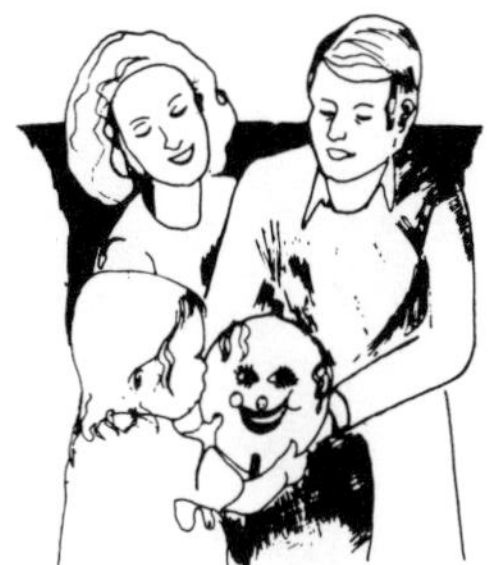

By <u>two years</u> of age, your baby should:

1. Point to at least one part of his body
   (eyes, feet, etc.) when you tell him
   to, without his seeing your lips.
2. Point to the right picture if you say
   "where's the cat" (or dog, or man, or
   horse) without his seeing your lips.
3. Give you a toy when you ask him to,
   or put a block on the table or chair
   when you ask him to, without his
   seeing your lips.

If your baby never does these things,

TELL THE BABY'S
DOCTOR ABOUT IT.

What you should be doing:

1. Read simple books to him and ask him
   "where's the kitty," and point out
   the pictures.
2. Ask him to put things in certain
   places: "Put the dolly on the chair,"
   "Put the ball under the table."
3. Talk, talk, talk to him about every-
   thing he plays with or sees.

These first two years are the most important years in your baby's life. Give him
all the attention and love you can.

Appendix **12–C**

Information Contained in Instructional Pamphlet Given to Nurses

**NURSES' ROLE IN
NEONATAL HEARING SCREENING
AT THE
READING HOSPITAL AND MEDICAL CENTER**

This pamphlet is designed as a guideline. If you have a question concerning any phase of completing the high-risk register or the screening procedures, please feel free to call the Speech and Hearing Center (6694).

It is only through the support of the nursing staff that the Neonatal Hearing Screening Program at The Reading Hospital and Medical Center can be a success. Thank you all for your cooperation.

Elca Swigart, Ph.D.
Coordinator
Neonatal Hearing Screening Program

INTERVIEWING THE MOTHER

Question 1–A. "Do you know any of the baby's relatives who now have a
   hearing loss that started before the age of 5 years?"

When you ask the first question, there are two important parts:

1. The loss occurred *before* the age of 5
2. The relative *still has* the hearing loss

Considerations:

If the mother doesn't know exactly when it started, but says "at a very
young age," count it as a hearing loss.

If the mother doesn't know whether or not they still have the loss, count
it as a hearing loss.

If the mother says that the relative's hearing is okay now, do not count it
as a hearing loss.

Question 1–B. (a) Who were they?

Please be sure to record the relationship of the relative to the baby. Record
only siblings, parents, grandparents, aunts, uncles, and first cousins.

Question 1–B. (b) Do you know what caused the loss?

The reason for the hearing loss in a relative is very important if the mother
knows. This information helps us determine hereditary factors. The loss
could be the result of childhood illness, fever, or trauma, or it may have
been present at birth. Do not count hearing loss as a result of acquired
disease, fever, or trauma in infancy or childhood.

Question 1–B. (c) What makes you think the onset of the hearing loss was
   before age 5 years?

The answer to this question helps us determine in a more precise manner
when the loss occurred. It also gives an indication of the reliability of the
mother's information.

Question 1–B. (d) Did he or she wear a hearing aid before the age of 5 years?

(e) Did he or she attend a special school for the deaf?

(f) Did he or she have a speech problem?

The answers to these questions help us determine the severity of the relative's hearing loss.

Question 2. "During your pregnancy, did you have Three-day measles, German measles, rubella, or a rash with a fever?"

Each of the perinatal infections (TORCH) may contribute to hearing loss.
We have become overconfident about perinatal rubella, believing that the
rubella vaccine solved all the problems. However, cases of rubella related
deafness in infants have been reported in recent years. Another important
fact to be considered is that the rubella virus lives a long time. Two deaf
infants have been reportedly born to mothers who had contracted rubella
prior to conception. There are also reports of positive cultures obtained in
children as late as 4 to 6 months postpartum. Other common occurring
sequelae of perinatal rubella are psychomotor and mental retardation, cataracts, and heart disease. Therefore, because of the long life of the rubella

virus and its severe effects, special attention is given to assessing its occurrence during pregnancy.

Although we are most concerned about the effects during the first trimester, count this as a risk if it occurs during any trimester. In addition, count an unnamed rash only if it were accompanied by a fever. Do not count chicken pox or roseola.

Question 3. "During your pregnancy, were you around anyone who had Three-day measles, German measles, rubella, or a rash with a fever?"

Sometimes an individual can contract a virus with manifestations so mild that he is unaware of having them. Therefore, we ask if the mother has been around someone who has had Three-day measles, German measles, rubella, or a rash with a fever. Count measles and any unnamed rash with a fever (do not include chicken pox or roseola) during any trimester as a risk.

Question 4. "Do you have any reason to be concerned about your baby's hearing?"

If there is any reason that the parent is concerned about the baby's hearing, a Crib-o-gram should be administered.

Question 5. "What pediatrician or clinic will be caring for your baby when he or she leaves the hospital?"

It is important to know who the pediatrician is who will be caring for the baby after he or she leaves the hospital because all reports concerning hearing will be sent to the physician.

AFTER THE INTERVIEW

1. Place a check in the first line of the high-risk register indicating whether or not there is a family history of childhood hearing impairments.
2. Give the mother the pamphlet concerning hearing.

THE HIGH-RISK REGISTER

The box containing the high-risk register is of vital importance in the tabulation of results. Please put a checkmark by *all* questions. When the audiologist or an audiological assistant tabulates the data or puts the information into the computer for later tabulation, he cannot guess at the results if there is no mark in either the "yes" or "no" columns.

CRIB-O-GRAM SCREENING

If there are one or more checks in the "yes" column of the high-risk register, administer a Crib-o-gram. The procedure for administering the Crib-o-gram is on the Crib-o-gram chart.

Then check either "PASS" or "REFER," and record the cursor number, the date, and your initials. The date may be later used to determine the chronological age at the time of testing. Your initials and the pediatrician's are helpful if there are any questions concerning the child or the testing procedure.

Finally, if there is a check by "REFER," call the Speech and Hearing Department and request auditory brainstem response (ABR) testing. The audiologist will fill in all other information concerning ABR.

NEONATAL HEARING SCREENING RECORD

As you know, you record all responses on pressure sensitive paper. The white sheet should remain in the baby's folder, and the yellow sheet should be sent to the Speech and Hearing Department.

WHAT HAPPENS NEXT?

1. If the baby is *not at risk* in any category, *no further follow-up* is needed.

2. If the baby is *at risk* and the *Crib-o-gram is administered,* there are two avenues to follow:

   (a) If the baby *passes* the *Crib-o-gram,* no immediate action is taken. However, because some types of hearing loss may occur after birth in these high-risk children, a questionnaire to determine whether there are any hearing problems will be sent to the parents when the baby is approximately 1 year old.

   (b) If the baby does *not pass* the Crib-o-gram, ABR is administered before the baby leaves the hospital. This is a more sensitive test than the Crib-o-gram. We expect a certain number of babies who do not pass the Crib-o-gram to have normal hearing. The Crib-o-gram is a *screening* test and is intended to identify those babies who should receive more in-depth testing.

      (1) If the baby *passes ABR,* no follow-up is requested. However, a questionnaire to assess whether or not there are any hearing problems is still sent to the parents when the baby is approximately 1 year old.

      (2) If the baby *does not pass ABR,* he is followed closely by the audiologist until a more accurate estimate of his hearing can be made and habilitation begun if necessary.

      (3) If the baby leaves the hospital over the weekend and ABR has not been administered, he is recalled at 3 months of age for the test.

Appendix **12–D**

Letter to Pediatrician if Baby Failed Crib-o-gram Screening but Passed Subsequent ABR Screening

Child's name ___________________

Address ___________________

____

Date of Birth ___________________

Dear Dr. ___________________ :

The Neonatal Hearing Screening Program at The Reading Hospital and Medical Center involves babies included in a High-Risk Register. The above-mentioned baby is considered at risk for hearing loss due to ___________________ ___________________ .

This child did not pass the Crib-o-gram hearing screening on (date) ___________________ . However, subsequent Auditory Brainstem Response screening suggests that the hearing sensitivity falls within expected limits.

This child *passed the hearing screening* at this time.

Because hearing loss can occur in this high-risk group sometime after birth, it would be wise if the parents were advised to observe the baby's responses to auditory stimuli for the next few months. Guidelines are in the pamphlet concerning hearing that was given to the mother.

Sincerely,

Coordinator
Neonatal Hearing Screening Program

Appendix **12–E**

Letter to Pediatrician if Baby Failed Both Crib-o-gram and ABR Screening

Child's name _______________________

Address _______________________

____

Date of Birth _______________________

Dear Dr. _______________________ :

The Neonatal Hearing Screening Program at The Reading Hospital and Medical Center involves newborn babies included in a High-Risk Register. The abovementioned baby is considered at risk for hearing loss due to ____

____ .

The child did not pass the Crib-o-gram screening test. Subsequent Auditory Brainstem Response screening indicated that responses to click stimuli did not fall within expected limits.

It is recommended that this child be *re-evaluated* with Auditory Brainstem Response testing *in approximately 3 months*. This can be accomplished at The Reading Hospital Speech and Hearing Center, and an appointment has been tentatively set. The parents will be notified of this appointment. If, however, it is more convenient to have the ABR retest performed elsewhere, the hospital's Speech and Hearing Center would appreciate receiving a copy of the test results to complete the follow-up program.

Thank you for your cooperation.

Sincerely,

Coordinator
Neonatal Hearing Screening Program

Appendix **12–F**

Letter to Pediatrician if Baby Failed Crib-o-gram Screening and Mother and Baby Were Released From the Hospital Without ABR Screening

Child's name ____________________
Address ______________________

____
Date of Birth __________________

Dear Dr. __________________ :

The Neonatal Hearing Screening Program at The Reading Hospital and Medical Center involves babies included in a High-Risk Register. The above-mentioned baby is considered at risk for hearing loss due to ______________
____ .

The child *did not pass the Crib-o-gram screening test*. The child and mother were released from the hospital before Auditory Brainstem Response screening could be administered.

It is recommended that this child be *evaluated with Auditory Brainstem Response* in approximately *3 months*. This can be accomplished at The Reading Hospital Speech and Hearing Center, and an appointment has been tentatively set. The parents will be notified of this appointment. If, however, it is more convenient to have the ABR test performed elsewhere, the hospital's Speech and Hearing Center would appreciate receiving a copy of the test results to complete the follow-up program.

Thank you for your cooperation.

Sincerely,

Coordinator
Neonatal Hearing Screening Program

Appendix **12–G**

Letter to Parents Indicating Three-Month Appointment for Hearing Testing

Dear ______________________ :

Your baby had a hearing test several months ago, and we feel that a re-check is necessary at this time to make sure that he or she is hearing as well as possible.

Your baby is scheduled for an audiological re-evaluation on ___________ ______________________ at ______________________ . Should it be impossible for you to keep this appointment, please call 378-6694 to re-schedule it.

The test may take 45 minutes to 2 hours, depending on how quickly your baby falls asleep. The baby *must be asleep* for a portion of the evaluation. Please do what you can to make sure that the baby is tired when he reaches the hospital. This may include getting him up a little early or attempting to have him miss a nap. If at all possible, please attempt to keep him awake during the drive to the hospital. It would also be helpful if you can arrange his feeding schedule so that he can be fed at the hospital just prior to the test.

Thank you for your cooperation. If you have any questions, please feel free to contact the Speech and Hearing Center.

Sincerely,

Coordinator
Neonatal Hearing Screening Program

Appendix **12–H**

Letter to Physician if Baby Passed Three-Month Hearing Testing

Child's name _______________________
Address _______________________
____
Date of Birth _______________________

Dear Dr. _______________________ :

The abovementioned baby was listed in The Reading Hospital and Medical Center's High-Risk Register for hearing loss. This baby did not pass the Crib-o-gram screening and Auditory Brainstem Response screening shortly after birth. Re-evaluation on (date) _______________________
with ABR indicates that the child's responses fell within expected limits.

This child *passed the hearing testing* at this time.

Because hearing loss can occur in a high-risk group sometime after birth, it would be wise if parents were advised to continue to observe the baby's responses to auditory stimuli within the next few months. Guidelines are in the pamphlet concerning hearing that was given to the mother at the time of birth.

Sincerely,

Coordinator
Neonatal Hearing Screening Program

Appendix **12–I**

Letter to Pediatrician if Baby Did Not Pass the Three-Month Hearing Testing

Child's name _____________________
Address _____________________
____
Date of Birth _____________________

Dear Dr. __________________ :

The abovementioned baby was listed in the High-Risk Register for hearing loss at The Reading Hospital and Medical Center. This baby did not pass the initial Crib-o-gram screening or Auditory Brainstem Response screening shortly after birth.

The child was re-evaluated with Auditory Brainstem Response testing on (date) ___________________________ , and the responses did not fall within expected limits.

It is therefore recommended that this child *receive a complete auditory evaluation at 7 months of age.* We will be glad to test this child at the Speech and Hearing Center of The Reading Hospital, and an appointment has been tentatively set. The parents will be notified of this appointment. However, if it is more convenient to have the testing performed elsewhere, we would appreciate a copy of these test results to complete our follow-up program.

Thank you for your cooperation.

Sincerely,

Coordinator
Neonatal Hearing Screening Program

Appendix **12–J**

Letter to Pediatrician if Baby Passed Complete Audiological Evaluation

Child's name ____________________
Address ____________________

____
Date of Birth ____________________

Dear Dr. __________________ :

The abovementioned baby was included in a High-Risk Register for hearing loss at The Reading Hospital and Medical Center. The child's responses to hearing screening at birth and threshold testing at 3 months did not fall within expected limits.

Today, a complete audiological evaluation suggested that hearing sensitivity falls within normal limits.

This child *passed the hearing testing* at this time.

Because hearing loss can occur in a high-risk group sometime after birth, it would be wise if parents were advised to continue to observe the baby's responses to auditory stimuli within the next few months. Guidelines are in the pamphlet concerning hearing that was given to the mother at the time of birth.

Sincerely,

Coordinator
Neonatal Hearing Screening Program

Appendix 12–K

Letter to Pediatrician if Baby Is Suspected to Have a Mild Hearing Loss at the Seven-Month Audiological Evaluation

Child's name ______________________

Address ______________________

____

Date of Birth ______________________

Dear Dr. ______________________ :

The abovementioned baby was included in a High-Risk Register for hearing loss at The Reading Hospital and Medical Center. The child's responses to hearing screening at birth and threshold testing at 3 months did not fall within expected limits.

A complete audiological evaluation on (date) ______________________ suggests the possibility of a *mild hearing loss*. (Information on test results may be included here.)

It is recommended that the child *continue with audiological surveillance* until a more definite indication of his hearing sensitivity is obtained. An otological evaluation may add useful information in this case if it has not been previously obtained.

Sincerely,

Coordinator
Neonatal Hearing Screening Program

Appendix **12–L**

Letter to Pediatrician Indicating a Significant Hearing Loss

Child's name ___________________
Address _______________________
____
Date of Birth __________________

Dear Dr. ___________________ :

The abovementioned baby was included in a High-Risk Register for hearing loss at The Reading Hospital and Medical Center. The child's responses to auditory stimuli at birth and at 3 months did not fall within expected limits.

A complete audiological evaluation today suggests that the child may have a *significant hearing loss*.

It is recommended that the child be fitted with amplification as soon as medical clearance for a hearing aid is obtained. An otological evaluation is recommended if one has not already been obtained.

We will be glad to continue following this child at The Reading Hospital's Speech and Hearing Center. If, however, the parents have any doubts concerning the child's hearing abilities, they are encouraged to obtain a second opinion. If testing is performed elsewhere, we would appreciate a copy of the test results to complete our follow-up program.

If the parents wish to continue to receive services at The Reading Hospital's Speech and Hearing Center, a hearing aid evaluation will be scheduled as soon as possible, and the child will be referred to the Preschool Hearing-Impaired Program.

Thank you for your cooperation. If we can be of any service regarding this child or if you have any questions, please do not hesitate to call the Speech and Hearing Center at 378-6694.

Sincerely,

Coordinator
Neonatal Hearing Screening Program

Appendix 12–M

Form for Medical Clearance for Amplification

Baby's Name: _______________________________________

                                             Last   First

Address: _______________________________________

Date of Birth: _______________________________________

This child has received a medical examination of the ears, and medical clearance for the use of amplification is granted.

____

                      Physician's Signature

Date: _______________________________________

Appendix **12–N**

Letter to Parent Requesting the Completion and Return of the One-Year Questionnaire

Dear ________________________________ :
          (parent's name)

A few days after your baby was born, he or she was given a Crib-o-gram hearing screening test. To complete the "follow-up" portion of our hearing screening program, we would appreciate your answering the questions on the enclosed questionnaire. Please return the questionnaire in the enclosed stamped, self-addressed envelope as soon as possible.

If you are concerned about your baby's hearing, TELL THE BABY'S DOCTOR ABOUT IT. If there is still some question about the baby's hearing, you may contact the Speech and Hearing Center at The Reading Hospital and Medical Center (215) 378-6694 for a hearing check.

Thank you for your help in completing the "follow-up" portion of our hearing screening program.

                Sincerely,

                Coordinator
                Neonatal Hearing Screening Program

Appendix **12–O**

One-Year Questionnaire

Baby's Name ________________________ Date of Birth ____________________

Please answer the following questions and return them to Reading Hospital and Medical Center in the enclosed stamped, self-addressed envelope. Your help is appreciated in completing the "follow-up" portion of our hearing screening program.

How old is your baby now? . . . . ______ months

Has your baby had any ear infections? . . . . ☐Yes   ☐No

   If "yes," about how many? . . . . ____________

Has he or she taken medication for his or her ears?   ☐Yes   ☐No

Does your baby stir or awaken when he or she is sleeping quietly and someone talks or makes a loud sound?   ☐ Never   ☐ Seldom   ☐ Usually

Does your baby turn his or her head in the direction of an interesting sound?   ☐ Never   ☐ Seldom   ☐ Usually

Does your baby turn his or her head when his or her name is called and he or she cannot see you?   ☐ Never   ☐ Seldom   ☐ Usually

Does your baby repeat some of the sounds you make?   ☐ Never   ☐ Seldom   ☐ Usually

Do you feel that your baby has any hearing problem?   ☐Yes   ☐No

If you are concerned about your baby's hearing,

TELL THE BABY'S DOCTOR ABOUT IT.

If there is still some question about the baby's hearing, you may contact the Speech and Hearing Center at Reading Hospital and Medical Center (215) 378-6694, for a hearing check.

PLEASE RETURN THIS QUESTIONNAIRE
AS SOON AS POSSIBLE

Chapter 13

MODEL PROGRAM V
A High-Risk Register by Computerized Search of Birth Certificates

Utah Department of Health
Bureau of Communicative Disorders
Salt Lake City, Utah

Thomas M. Mahoney
John G. Eichwald

High-risk hearing screening in Utah is implemented by the Bureau of Communicative Disorders in the Division of Family Health Services of the Utah Department of Health. The Division is responsible for planning, promoting, and coordinating health services for mothers, infants, and children in Utah through consultative, contractual, and direct service provision. The Bureau has been providing speech, hearing, and language services to the children of Utah for more than 40 years. Consistent with the Division's purpose, Bureau goals emphasize early identification and intervention for the preschool child and service to population areas that are lacking local speech and hearing programs. Funding is primarily from the federal maternal and child health block grant to the states.

Mass newborn hearing screening began in Utah as a pilot project in 1967 and eventually included the behavioral screening of all newborns in seven hospitals throughout the state. In accordance with the 1974 supplementary statement of the Joint Committee on Infant Hearing and the proceedings of the Nova Scotia Conference on Early Identification (Mencher, 1975), the Bureau adopted a high-risk register in favor of mass newborn hearing screening. By 1976, a statewide risk register that addressed the original five high-risk criteria recommended by the Joint Committee was in effect. This program used a hospital maternal questionnaire designed to obtain accurate data with minimal hospital or professional participation. However, maximal effort with available resources resulted in a questionnaire return rate of approximately 50 percent of the total live birth population (Mahoney and Eichwald, 1979). It was thought that this limited return of questionnaires compromised the effectiveness of the program.

Beginning in 1978, the birth certificate became the initial screening device in Utah's high-risk hearing screening program. Its use had several immediate attractions. Most importantly, because the birth certificate is a legal mandate, a register based on this document would include almost all the state's live births. It was also obvious that such a register could be implemented with minimal effort, since an elaborate system of collecting birth information was already in place. Finally, it was realized that with the addition of a question concerning family history of hearing loss, virtually all the recommended risk criteria could be addressed by surveying the birth certificate, thus avoiding the need for a separate data collection and analysis system.

Initial optimism was tempered by knowledge that certain problems are reported to exist concerning the accuracy of birth certificate information (Green, Nelson, Gaylor, and Holson, 1979) and that permission to add a question to the birth certificate is extremely difficult to acquire. The first problem remains and will be discussed later in this chapter. The second problem was fortunately alleviated by the active cooperation of the director of the Utah Bureau of Health Statistics. In realizing the potential of this innovative program, he was instrumental in convincing the Health Statistics Advisory Committee to include the family history question on the official Utah birth certificate in 1978. Instrumental in this decision was the fact that the Bureau of Communicative Disorders already had in effect a successful high-risk hearing screening program. Since 1978, more than 280,000 live births have been screened for hearing impairment by computerized search of their birth certificates. The following section will detail the operational functions of this program, which are chronologically outlined in Fig. 13–1.

PROGRAM PROCEDURES

This section will highlight those aspects of the program important to its initial development and continued operation. Only currently operating procedures will be discussed, except when an explanation of earlier procedures is needed for clarification. It should

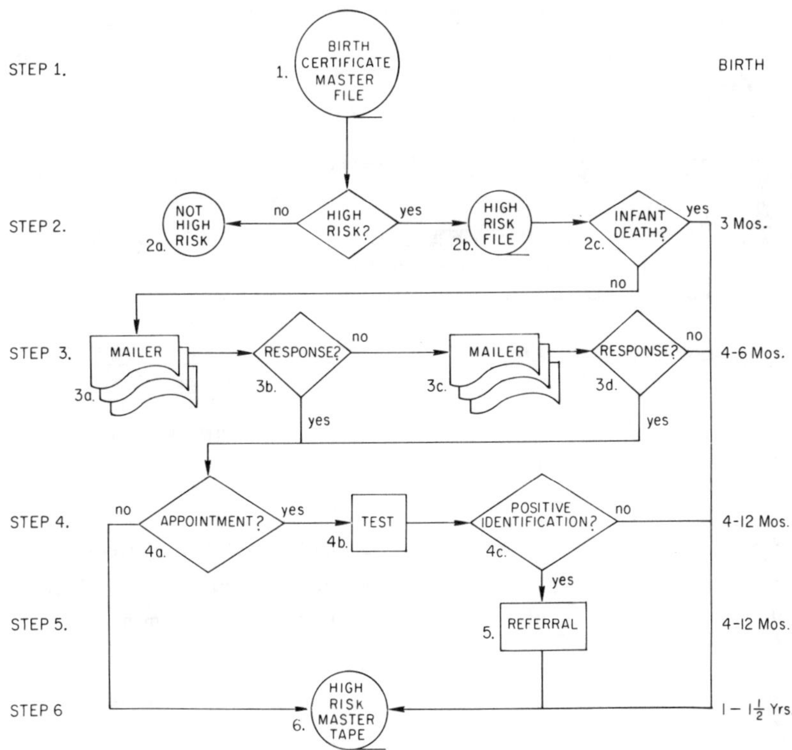

Figure 13–1. Chronological program flow chart. 1. Birth certificates completed in hospital. 2(a). Bureau of Health Statistics (BHS) purges non-high-risk certificates. 2(b). BHS generates high-risk (HR) file. 2(c). Infant deaths purged from file. 3(a). HR packet is generated and mailed by BHS computer process. 3(b). Appointment request card returned to Bureau of Communicative Disorders. 3(c). Non-responder receives second mailer after 2 months. 3(d). No response to second mailer results in closure. 4(a). Hearing screening appointments made upon request. 4(b). Audiological assessment made. 4(c). Positive identification determined. 5. Appropriate referral made. 6. Information updated onto HR master tape.

be realized that current program protocols have evolved from more than 7 years of experience with the birth certificate model. This process has involved a wide variety of procedural trial and error that has continued to the present time.

The Birth Certificate

The basic instrument for high-risk hearing screening in Utah is the official birth certificate, a legally mandatory document for all live births. Figure 13–2 highlights those portions of the document perti-

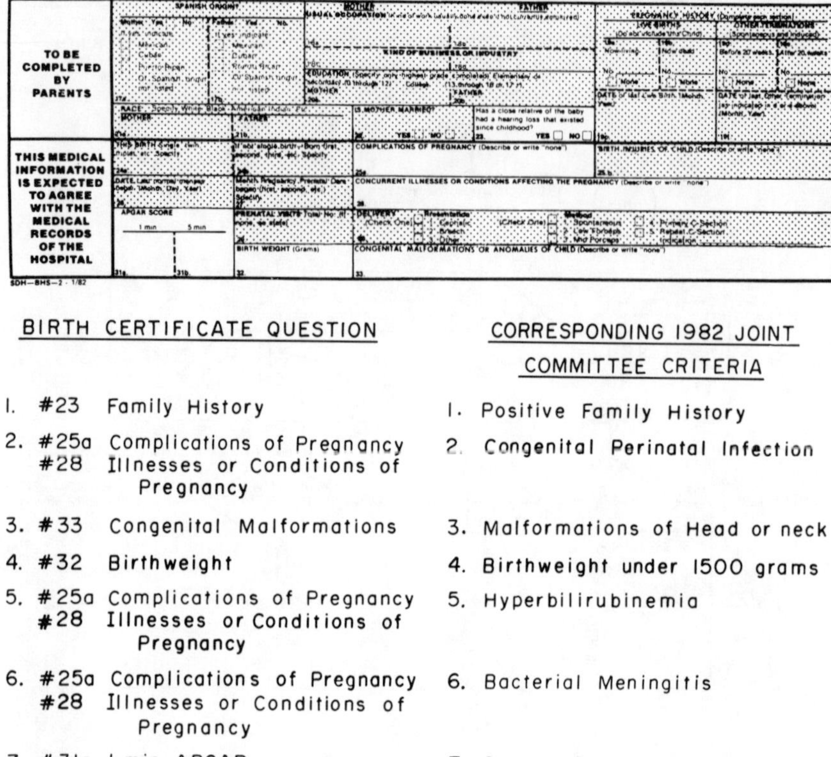

BIRTH CERTIFICATE QUESTION

CORRESPONDING 1982 JOINT
COMMITTEE CRITERIA

1. #23   Family History

1. Positive Family History

2. #25a Complications of Pregnancy
  #28   Illnesses or Conditions of
        Pregnancy

2. Congenital Perinatal Infection

3. #33   Congenital Malformations

3. Malformations of Head or neck

4. #32   Birthweight

4. Birthweight under 1500 grams

5. #25a Complications of Pregnancy
  #28   Illnesses or Conditions of
        Pregnancy

5. Hyperbilirubinemia

6. #25a Complications of Pregnancy
  #28   Illnesses or Conditions of
        Pregnancy

6. Bacterial Meningitis

7. #31a 1 min APGAR
  #31b 5 min APGAR

7. Severe Asphyxia

Figure 13–2. Utah birth certificates health information section, highlighting those portions pertinent to the high-risk program. Specific birth certificate questions and their corresponding 1982 Joint Committee recommended criteria are listed below the document.

nent to the high-risk program. Specific questions that relate to the risk criteria recommended by the 1982 Joint Committee are listed below the document.

The screening process begins with the completion of the birth certificate. All new parents are requested to answer the question concerning positive family history of hearing loss within several days following the birth of their child. They are instructed by hospital staff as to what constitutes a true positive family history. Other questions pertinent to high-risk factors are answered with information obtained from the hospital chart or the birth certificate worksheet. These include Apgar scores (a subjective numerical index of the newborn's condition at 1 and 5 minutes after birth) and birthweight. Complications of pregnancy, illnesses or conditions affecting the pregnancy, and congenital anomalies are written directly on the certificate by the physician, attending nurse or midwife, or other hospital staff.

Birth certificates are accumulated by the hospitals, sent to the county registrar for recording, and are subsequently mailed to the State Bureau of Health Statistics. There, within 90 days of the birth, the certificates are data reduced by keypunch onto a monthly birth computer tape. This data collection involves the expertise of a nosologist who supervises the coding of all hand-written descriptive items according to the International Classification of Diseases (ICD) codes. A monthly high-risk file, which includes infants who fail any one or more of the risk items, is generated from the master birth tape. This file, in conjunction with a computer-automated mailing process, is used to notify parents 4 to 6 months post partum. Source documents (individual computer-generated patient data records) and an alphabetical listing of high-risk infants are generated monthly.

Parental Notification

The first mailing to parents of risk infants contains three types of information: an explanation of the program, a hearing developmental check list, and a postage-paid, addressed parental response card. As shown in Figure 13–3, various parental options are on this card. These include a request for a screening appointment, an indication that the baby has already been tested or will be tested, no parental concern, and additional comments. The risk criteria for which the infant was placed on the register are computer printed on the card. The parents of babies placed at risk for family history also receive a special notice indicating what constitutes a true family history of hearing loss. In an attempt to reduce a high false-positive response to this question, parents who answered the family history question incorrectly are requested to write "is not at risk" on the card and return it to the Bureau.

The records of infants whose parents are unable to be contacted because of incorrect address are closed to the program. Parents who do not respond to the first mailing are sent a second mailing in 2 months. The second mailing contains the same materials as originally sent, plus a special cover card that restates that the baby has a higher than normal chance of hearing loss. No response to the second mailing results in no further contact and closure.

Screening and Diagnosis

Parents requesting state screening services have a choice of one of five audiology centers or one of eight itinerant sites that hold clinics three times a year.

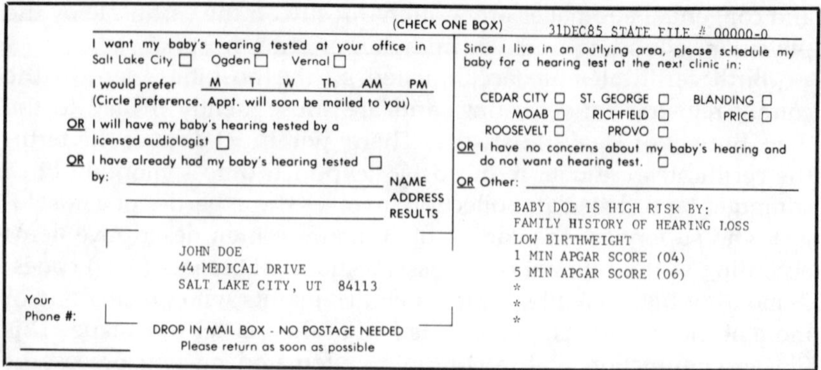

Figure 13–3. The parental response card. This postage-paid card contains computer-printed information concerning parental address, date of birth, state file number, and high risk criteria. It is automatically enclosed in the high-risk packet and mailed to the parents.

Audiology Center Screening

At the audiology centers, appointments are typically scheduled within 1 month of receiving the parental response card. Appointments are confirmed by phone the day preceding the scheduled visit. A broken first appointment results in a closure of the infant's record. The parents bring to their appointment a complete history questionnaire that was mailed with the appointment letter. The history questionnaire includes a general developmental profile from a chronological check list. A brief parental interview verifies gestational age, confirms the high-risk condition, provides information on auditory responses observed in the home, updates medical history, and supplies other pertinent information.

The screening protocol is designed to enable a sole audiologist to obtain enough information in a one-half hour session to pass or fail an infant. Threshold data are not sought. Pass-fail criteria are based on published norms modified by clinical experience and are designed to identify those infants who do not have hearing adequate for normal speech and language development. Because the testing involves a sound field procedure, monaural hearing status is not specifically determined. Experience has shown, however, that significant unilateral loss can often be identified by qualitative analysis of the responses.

The sound field behavioral hearing assessment uses visual reinforcement procedures in a two-room sound isolation suite. The infant is seated on the parent's lap facing the audiologist in the control room. Two loudspeakers are located at ear level, 1.5 meters from the infant and at 45-degree angles to both sides of the infant's midline of vision. The visual reinforcers are commercially produced animated toy animals that light up in dark enclosures. They are placed on top of each loudspeaker. Hearing screening begins with a conditioning paradigm consisting of 50 dB HL live voice with simultaneous visual reinforcement. After conditioning, a 100 percent visual reinforcement schedule is used in conjunction with a descending order of stimulus presentation. The stimuli include live voice and high pass filtered live voice (cut off frequency at 2000 Hz with a 48 dB per octave roll off). Localization in both directions at 20 dB is considered passing for a 4- to 5-month-old infant, whereas those 6 months or older are required to respond at 15 dB HL. Response requirements for premature infants are adjusted for gestational age. A sudden voice burst or white noise from 65 to 75 dB HL is used to elicit an aural-palpebral reflex or startle response. The screening session is concluded following acoustic immittance assessment and appropriate parental counseling.

Itinerant Clinic Screening

A number of parents prefer to bring their infant into one of the itinerant clinics in rural areas of the state. In this case, the parents may contact their local public health office directly for scheduling, or they may request scheduling coordination through the Bureau's central office. Two weeks prior to a scheduled clinic, appointment letters are sent to parents. Names, addresses, and phone numbers of the high-risk respondents are simultaneously sent to the local public health nurse. A few days prior to the scheduled clinic, the nurse phones the parent to confirm the screening appointment.

Screening protocols at the itinerant clinics are adjusted for the lack of sound-isolated environment. The infants are usually several months older (about 7 to 9 months of age) than those seen at the regional audiology centers. Hearing sensitivity is estimated by observing localization responses to calibrated sound field noise-makers or portable visual reinforcement hearing screening systems, both described in Northern and Downs (1984). Acoustic immittance is performed using portable equipment. Infants who fail itinerant clinic screening are either referred to an audiology center for diagnostic testing or are rescreened 1 to 3 months later at the local health department. The time frame and location for rescreening or diagnostic testing are based on availability of resources, extent of suspected loss, status of the middle ears, and the need for medical follow-up.

Diagnostic Testing

Diagnostic hearing testing at the audiology centers emphasizes detailed threshold search using air- and bone-conducted pure tone or narrowband stimuli. Auditory evoked potential evaluations are performed on all infants with suspected sensorineural hearing loss or difficult-to-test children. This is preferably performed when middle ear function is documented to be normal by acoustic immittance measures.

Referral and Follow-up

Once a hearing loss is documented, the policy of the Bureau is to refer the infant to other resources whenever possible. The infant's health care provider is notified at this point and is instrumental in medical management of middle ear pathology or medical clearance for amplification. If parents have adequate personal financial resources or third party coverage, referral is made to other resources for continued audiological services. As soon as possible after confirmation of significant hearing loss, habilitative referral is made to the statewide Parent–Infant Program (PIP), operated by the Utah Schools for the Deaf and Blind. This program affords early home intervention for hearing-impaired infants on a weekly basis and hearing aid management without charge to the parents (Clark and Watkins, 1978). Parent advisors teach effective methods of stimulating language and speech skills at as early an age as possible. Aural or total communication may be emphasized, depending on team assessment, individual needs, and parental preference.

Trial amplification is based on behavioral and electrophysiological data. Auditory brainstem response–assisted hearing aid evaluations may be performed, as described by Mahoney (1985). The PIP hearing aid loan bank is used for trial periods for amplification. A parent advisor begins training in effective hearing aid use as soon as the hearing aids have been fitted. Once sufficient hearing aid use is established, a clinical hearing aid evaluation is performed by the managing audiologist. Information on the child's auditory responsiveness from the home setting is incorporated into this evaluation, and the combination of clinical and observational data helps determine appropriate hearing aid purchase. The Bureau of Communicative Disorders purchases hearing aids for infants of financially needy parents.

Follow-up audiological services are usually provided by PIP or private audiologists. The Bureau routinely follows children for whom it has purchased hearing aids. Infants with significant developmental delays or other handicapping conditions are referred to either a developmental nurse at the local health department or to Handicapped Children's Services within the Division of Family Health Services. Genetic counseling is provided by the Division and is recommended to parents of infants with family history of hearing loss or hearing loss of unknown etiology. Psychological counseling is also available to help parents cope with having a hearing-impaired child.

Parental response and clinical and habilitative information are recorded on each infant's high-risk source document. By 18 months of age, at the latest, all data are keypunched into the master high-risk file for the year that the child was born. Annual statistical reports are generated from this file, which serves as the major data bank for program evaluation, upgrading, and reporting requirements.

The cost of the high-risk program, not including testing, is slightly more than one United States dollar per live birth. This includes the cost to generate and run the computer program, the printing, the postage, and the necessary staff salaries. Screening and testing are provided without charge to parents from general Bureau funds. The Bureau is required by the state legislature, however, to bill insurance and other third party payers, when applicable.

RESULTS

As shown in Figure 13–4, the high-risk hearing screening program has undergone several changes in the last 7 years. At the onset of the program, the high-risk criteria included only positive family history, low birthweight, and 5-minute Apgar scores of less than 7. In 1981, a 1-minute Apgar score of less than 5 was included as a risk item. With the advent of ICD coding of certificates in 1983, defects of head or neck, congenital perinatal infection, and bacterial meningitis were also incorporated. In a move to improve program efficiency, Apgar scores were restricted in 1984 to include scores less than 6 at 5 minutes and less than 4 at 1 minute.

Of 205,571 live births from 1978 to 1982, 18,228 (8.9 percent) were determined to be at risk for hearing loss by computer search of their birth certificates. As illustrated in Figure 13–5a, most of these infants were classified high-risk by one factor only: 10,619 (58.3 percent) by family history, 5346 (29.3 percent) by Apgar scores, and 621 (3.4 percent) by low birthweight. More than 8 percent were high-risk by two factors: 985 (5.4 percent) by both Apgar score(s) and birthweight, 438 (2.4 percent) by both family history and Apgar score(s), and 128 (0.7 percent) by both family history and birthweight. A total of 91 (0.5 percent) infants were at risk by all three factors (shaded area). The total occurrence of each risk factor in this population, that is, alone or in combination with all other factors, is illustrated in Figures 13–5b, c,

1978	FH	BW	AP5 (0-6)				
1979	FH	BW	AP5 (0-6)				
1980	FH	BW	AP5 (0-6)				
1981	FH	BW	AP5 (0-6)	API (0-4)			
1982	FH	BW	AP5 (0-6)	API (0-4)			
1983	FH	BW	AP5 (0-6)	API (0-4)	ENT	INF	MNG
1984	FH	BW	AP5 (0-5)	API (0-3)	ENT	INF	MNG

KEY

FH -POSITIVE FAMILY HISTORY
BW -BIRTHWEIGHT UNDER 1500 GRAMS
AP5 -FIVE MINUTE APGAR SCORE
API -ONE MINUTE APGAR SCORE
ENT -DEFECTS OF HEAD AND NECK
INF -CONGENITAL PERINATAL INFECTIONS
MNG-BACTERIAL MENINGITIS

Figure 13–4. A chronological order of the program's high-risk selection criteria from 1978–1984.

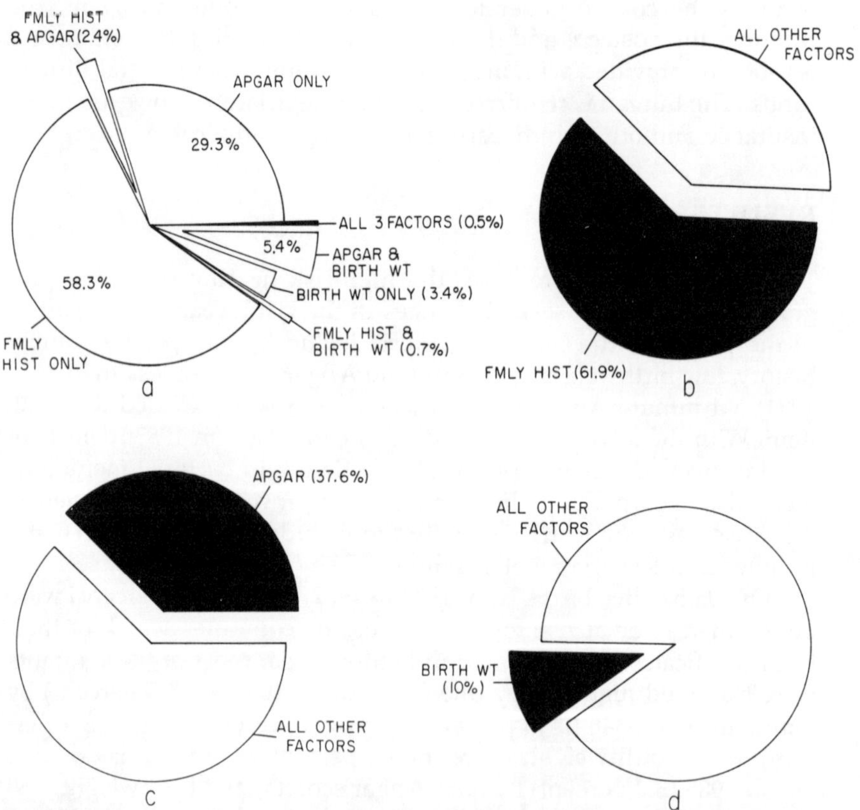

Figure 13–5. Analysis of risk criteria that identified 18,228 at-risk newborns from 1978–1982. Part a illustrates the occurrence of each risk factor when found in isolation and when it appeared in conjunction with other criteria. Parts b, c, and d illustrate the total occurrence of positive family history, low Apgar scores, and low birthweight, respectively.

d. Almost two thirds of the high-risk infants had positive family history of hearing loss, more than one third had low Apgar score(s), and 10 percent had birthweight under 1500 gm.

In 1983, the computer program was updated to include defects of head or neck, congenital perinatal infection, and bacterial meningitis. Due to the ICD coding procedures required to obtain this information from the birth certificates, these three are referred to as Type II high-risk criteria. Figure 13–6 illustrates a composite high-risk item analysis of 3952 at-risk infants born in 1983, which includes Type II data. Most of these infants were at risk by only one factor: 2037 (51.5 percent) by family history, 1486 (37.1 percent) by Apgar score(s), 86 (2.2 percent) by Type II, and 63 (1.6 percent) by birthweight. In total, 285 infants were at risk by two factors, 12 (0.3 percent) had three high-risk factors, and only one (0.03 percent) infant was at risk by all four criteria. It should be noted that the inclusion of Type II risk criteria only increased the total high-risk population by slightly more than 2 percent.

The high-risk master tape is annually updated by the Bureau of Health Statistics. Due to an inherent delay in obtaining habilitative information, it is only possible to present 5 years of complete patient data at this time. Figure 13–7 illustrates the outcome of a total of 205,571 live births from 1978 to 1982. Of these, 18,228 (8.9 percent) infants were classified at risk by the criteria listed in Figure 13–4. After purging for infant deaths, informational and appointment request packets were mailed to 93.9 percent of the high-risk infants' parents. Approximately one half (50.9 percent) of the parents responded to the mailers during these years. Of the 8721 mailers returned, about one half (51.3 percent) requested screening appointments at the Bureau. From 4476 appointment requests received, 3181 (71.1 percent) infants had their hearing screened by the Bureau. Of these, 891 (28 percent) were found to have middle ear involvement. Of all infants known to be screened by any provider, 68 (1.8 percent) were identified with sensorineural impairment.

Risk Factor(s)	1 RISK FACTOR				2 RISK FACTORS						3 FACTORS		ALL FACTORS	TOTAL HIGH RISK
	FH	AP	II	BW	AP BW	FH AP	AP II	FH BW	FH II	BW II	FH AP BW	AP BW II	FH AP BW II	
Number of Births	2037	1468	86	63	170	87	11	10	6	1	9	3	1	3,952
Percent of Births	51.5	37.1	2.2	1.6	4.3	2.2	0.28	0.25	0.15	0.03	0.23	0.08	0.03	100.0%

Figure 13–6. High-risk item analysis of 3952 at-risk infants born in 1983.

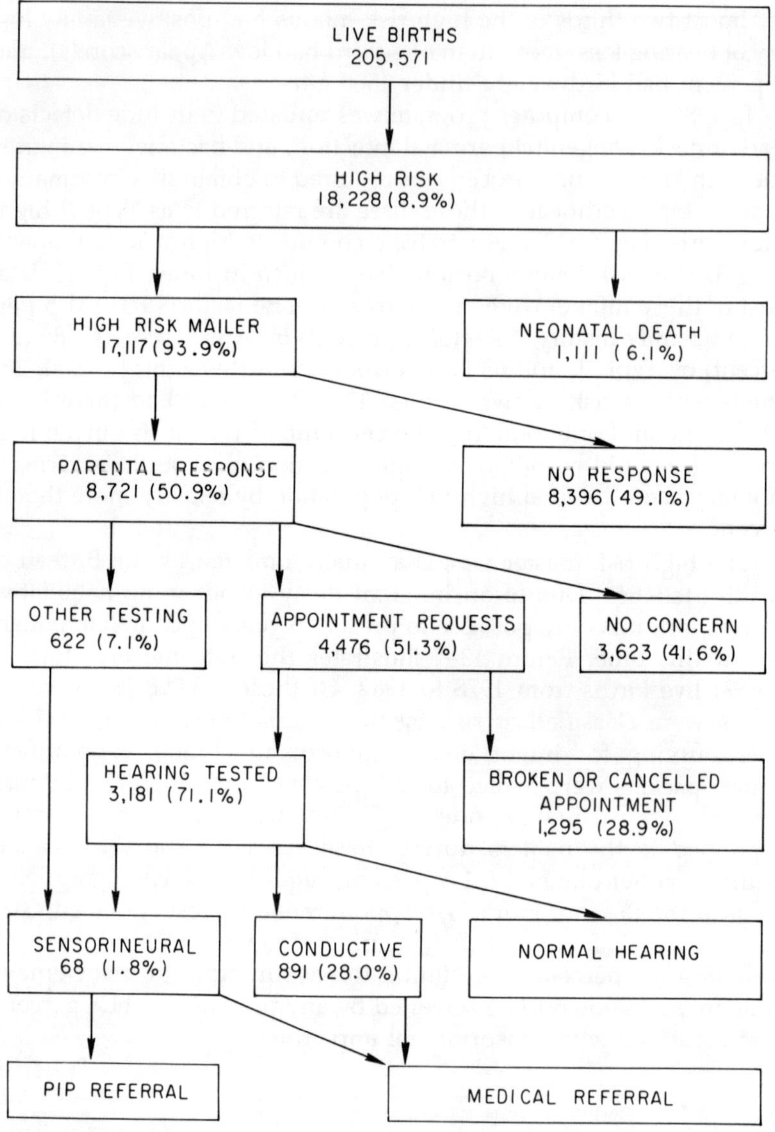

Figure 13–7. High-risk patient flow chart for 205,571 live births from 1978–1982.

Figure 13–8 represents the high-risk criteria instrumental in the identification of 85 sensorineural hearing-impaired infants from the program's inception in 1978 to the time of this writing. As illustrated in Figure 13–8a, the majority of the hearing-impaired infants were at risk by only one factor: 33 (38.8 percent) by family history, 23 (27.1

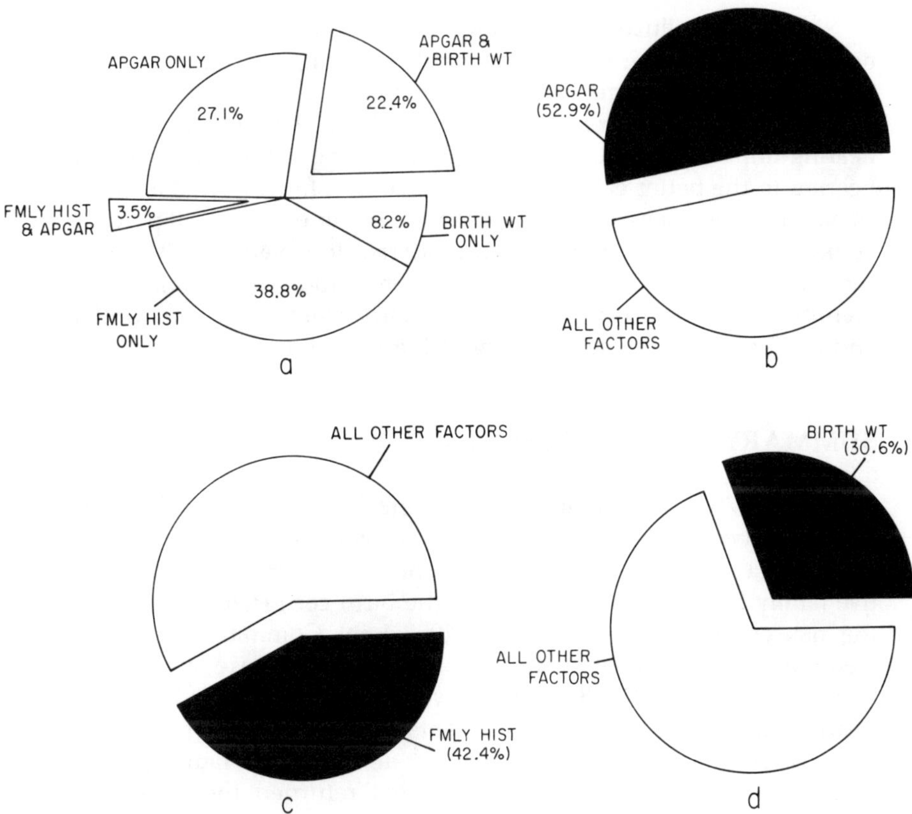

Figure 13–8. Analysis of risk criteria responsible for the identification of 85 sensorineural hearing-impaired infants from 1978 to the time of this writing. Part a illustrates the occurrence of each risk factor when found in isolation and when it appeared in conjunction with other criteria. Parts b, c, and d illustrate the total occurrence of low Apgar scores, positive family history, and low birthweight, respectively.

percent) by Apgar, and 7 (8.2 percent) by low birthweight. The remainder were high-risk by two risk factors: 19 (22.4 percent) by both low Apgar and low birthweight, and 3 (3.5 percent) by both family history and low Apgar. To date, no infants have been identified as having sensorineural hearing loss on the basis of more than two factors, nor by any Type II criteria. The total occurrence of each risk factor in this group is illustrated in Figures 13–8b, c, d. It is seen that 45 (52.9 percent) hearing-impaired infants were at risk by Apgar alone or in combination with another criterion, 36 (42.4 percent) by family history either alone or in combination, and 26 (30.6 percent) by total low birthweight.

Figure 13–9 illustrates the degree of impairment of 85 sensorineural hearing-impaired infants identified during the reporting period. These data are reported on the basis of degree of hearing impairment in the better ear. Note that two (2.3 percent) of the 85 hearing-impaired infants had unilateral hearing losses, with normal hearing in the better ear. Nine (10.6 percent) infants were diagnosed as having a mild sensorineural loss in the better ear, 17 (20.0 percent) as moderate, 10 (11.8 percent) as moderate to severe, 27 (31.8 percent) as severe, and 20 (23.5 percent) as profound. The average age of identification of sensorineural hearing impairment was 7.6 months, and the average first use of amplification was at 9.8 months.

SUMMARY AND DISCUSSION

From 1978 to 1984, more than a quarter of a million live births in Utah have been screened for hearing loss by computerized search of their birth certificates. By the addition of a question concerning positive family history of hearing loss to the birth certificate, virtually all the risk criteria suggested by the 1982 Joint Committee on Infant Hearing have been screened in this population. Of those infants born between 1978 and 1982, 8.9 percent were determined to be at risk for hearing impairment, and their parents were sent high-risk notices and materials outlining normal auditory development. During this 5-year period, more than half the parents returned their response cards, and more than half of those responding requested hearing screening appointments. Significantly, of those newborns screened, 28 percent were found to have middle ear involvement, and 1.8 percent were identified with sensorineural hearing impairment. This early identification allowed for the fitting of amplification, when indicated, at an average of 9.8 months of age. It is notable that almost one of three high-risk infants screened were determined to have hearing loss or middle ear involvement or both. Clearly, this reflects the high-

Degree of Loss	Normal with Unilateral Loss	Mild	Moderate	Mod–severe	Severe	Profound
Number of Infants	2	9	17	10	27	20
Percent of Hearing Impaired	2.3%	10.6%	20.0%	11.8%	31.8%	23.5%

Figure 13–9. Degree of impairment of 85 sensorineural hearing-impaired infants.

risk status of the target population and the high identification sensitivity of the program protocol.

Positive family history of hearing loss was reported on almost two thirds of the high-risk birth certificates, making it the most frequently reported risk criterion. The fact that positive family history occurred in more than 40 percent of the sensorineural hearing-impaired infants suggests that it also is a very sensitive predictor of significant hearing loss.

More than one third of the at-risk infants had low Apgar scores. This was the most frequently reported risk condition in infants identified with sensorineural hearing loss, suggesting that, as used in this program, Apgar may be the single most powerful predictor of hearing loss in the newborn population. At the inception of the program, specific Apgar scores were unestablished as high-risk indicators of hearing loss, leading us to intentionally widen the cut-off criteria for investigative purposes. If only scores from 0 to 3 were considered indicators of risk, as is currently recommended by the Joint Committee, 11 of 21 (53 percent) of the sensorineural hearing-impaired infants identified by Apgar alone would not have appeared on the register.

Less than 10 percent of the high-risk population had birthweight below 1500 gms, and, in 1983, only 2.7 percent had a positive response to one or more of the pregnancy or congenital anomaly questions (Type II risk factors). Although almost one third of the sensorineural hearing-impaired population had low birthweight, only 8.2 percent were identified by low birthweight alone. Not one infant identified with sensorineural loss had a positive Type II response. This does not infer that perinatal infections, congenital anomalies, and meningitis are not important risk criteria. It indicates, rather, that the birth certificate is probably not a sensitive register for these three conditions and that other means should probably be used to assess these criteria.

In spite of the above, the birth certificate remains a very efficient tool in effecting a statewide newborn high-risk hearing screening register. Most states have years of experience in effectively collecting and analyzing birth information, and compliance is ensured by legal mandate. Also, it is important to note that in Utah there is a 99 percent completion rate for questions treating family history, Apgar scores, and birthweight. In that other questions addressing the additional Joint Committee criteria require a written response, they are often left blank and their accuracy has been questioned by other investigators (Green et al., 1979).

Other factors that tend to lower overall program efficiency include parents who are unable to be contacted, reduced parental response and concern, unkept appointments, and false-positive family history responses. These all contribute to a limited number of at-risk infants screened from the original high-risk target population, and, consequently, vigorous attempts have been made to improve in these areas. Parental response to the high-risk notification mailer has increased from 25 percent in 1979 to almost 65 percent in 1983, primarily due to heightened public awareness and the institution of a second follow-up mailer in 1980. The rather high number of parents who report a lack of concern for their babies' hearing status is not overly concerning, in that it probably reflects increased awareness of normal auditory development as a result of the educational materials included in the mailer. The number of unkept screening appointments has significantly dropped with the institution of a telephone call reminder. The estimated 50 percent false-positive response to the family history question on the birth certificate has been approached in various ways. These include hospital staff giving specific instructions to assist parents in answering the question, the inclusion of a special insert in the mailer describing true family history of hearing loss and, more recently, a telephone contact verifying the family history prior to making the screening appointment.

In addition to efforts to improve program efficiency, the hearing screening protocol itself is frequently evaluated for overall effectiveness. Recently, the use of high-pass filtered speech was compared with warble tone and narrowband stimuli in an effort to improve the ability of the procedure to identify high-frequency hearing loss. Preliminary findings suggest narrowband noise may be preferable, because it elicits repeatable localization responses, at or near threshold levels, that offer more definitive high-frequency information. Pass-fail criteria under investigation are conditioned bilateral localization responses to live voice at 15 dB HL and to 500 Hz and 4000 Hz narrowband noises at 20 dB nHL. It appears that narrowband noise may replace the 2000 Hz high-pass filtered speech portion of the hearing screening protocol outlined earlier in this chapter.

The primary goal of screening is to identify as many abnormal infants as possible in a target population (sensitivity), while at the same time correctly classifying the normal infants (specificity). If the commonly quoted prevalence of significant sensorineural hearing loss is accurate, that is, one in 1000 to 2000 live births, it is expected that from 20 to 40 of these infants would be born annually in Utah. Therefore, a 100 percent effective screening program would have identified 100 to 200 infants with significant sensorineural hearing loss between 1978 and 1982. In actuality, only 68 sensorineural losses were identified. In examining rationale for this discrepancy, several possibilities occur. First, restricted high-risk registers are reported to identify only 50 to 80 percent of the total deaf population (Altman, 1968; Bergstrom, Hemenway, and Downs, 1971; Feinmesser, Tell, and

Levi, 1982; Salmivalli, Suonpaa, Johansson, and Jauhiainen, 1980). Second, risk registors geared for very early identification will likely miss children with progressive hearing loss. Third, an unknown number of hearing-impaired infants are probably overlooked due to the previously discussed insensitivity of the birth certificate to Type II criteria. Finally, identification rate is directly proportional to the number of at-risk infants who are actually screened, which is limited by the many programmatic factors already described. In spite of these limitations, the program has a 1.8 percent identification rate of sensorineural hearing loss in high-risk infants known to be tested (Fig. 13-6). This compares favorably with the incidence reported to be expected in a high-risk newborn population (Joint Committee on Infant Hearing Screening, 1972).

In conclusion, the Utah high-risk hearing screening program is believed to be a worthwhile and cost-effective public health endeavor. It has educated thousands of parents and health care professionals about the importance of early identification of hearing loss and, with limited funds, has been instrumental in identifying hundreds of hearing-impaired infants at a very early age. Early identification is known to decrease the cost of special services for hearing-impaired children and to permit increased tax revenues from habilitated hearing-impaired workers and serves to improve their general quality of life. High-risk hearing screening by birth certificate has proved to be an effective method to screen for hearing loss in large general newborn populations.

ACKNOWLEDGMENTS

The authors thank John Brockart, director of the Utah Bureau of Health Statistics, and his staff who were instrumental in the development of this program. Additionally, we thank Ronda Condie for her kind assistance in data compilation and Pamela Sanford for her patience throughout the preparation of this chapter.

REFERENCES

Altman, M. M. (1968). *Methods of early detection of hearing loss: Final report.* Haifa, Israel: H. Rambam Government Hospital.

Bergstrom, L., Hemenway, W. G., and Downs, M. P. (1971). A high-risk registry to find congenital deafness. *Otolaryngologic Clinics of North America, 4,* 369–399.

Clark, T. C., and Watkins, S. (1978). *The SKI*HI Model: Programming for hearing-impaired infants through amplification and home intervention.* Logan, UT: Utah State University.

Feinmesser, M., Tell, L., and Levi, H. (1982). Follow-up of 40,000 infants screened for hearing defect. *Audiology, 21*, 197–203.

Green, H. G., Nelson, C. J., Gaylor, D. W., and Holson, J. F. (1979). Accuracy of birth certificate data for detecting facial cleft defects in Arkansas children. *Cleft Palate Journal, 16*, 167–170.

Joint Committee on Infant Hearing Screening (1972). Supplementary statement. *ASHA, 16*(3), 160.

Joint Committee on Infant Hearing (1982). Position statement. *ASHA, 24*(12), 1017–1018.

Mahoney, T. (1985). Auditory brainstem response hearing aid application. In J. Jacobson (Ed.), *The auditory brainstem response.* San Diego: College-Hill Press.

Mahoney, T., and Eichwald, J. (1979). Newborn high-risk hearing screening by maternal questionnaire. *Journal of the American Auditory Society, 5*, 41–45.

Mencher, G. T. (1975). Nova Scotia conference on the early identification of hearing loss: A review. *Human Communication Journal, 3*, 5–20.

Northern, J., and Downs, M. (1984). *Hearing in children* (3rd ed.). Baltimore: Williams and Wilkins.

Salmivalli, A., Suonpaa, J., Johansson, R., and Jauhiainen, T. (1980). Early detection and identification of congenital hearing defects. *Suomen Laakarilehti, 8.*

Chapter 14

MODEL PROGRAM VI
An Infant Hearing Assessment Foundation SYNAP Program

Methodist Hospital
Indianapolis, Indiana

Alan Salamy
Christina Weyland

The Infant Hearing Assessment Foundation (IHAF) is a nonprofit organization directed toward the detection of hearing loss in infancy. The IHAF promotes early identification of hearing deficits through the implementation of infant screening programs. By providing a special-purpose computer (the Synap I) for the recording of auditory brainstem responses (ABRs) and arranging for local, public service volunteers (e.g., Telephone Pioneers, American Legion, Lions) to conduct the tests and carry out the program, the Foundation offers cost-effective, large-scale hearing screening to participating hospitals. In this way, the Foundation contributes to a valuable community function and thereby achieves its objectives.

COMPONENTS OF AN IHAF PROGRAM

Each IHAF Program is composed of several interacting components: (1) a hospital and staff that recognize a need for newborn hearing screening; (2) a professional, typically an audiologist, to direct the program and interface with the hospital staff (including physicians, nurses, administration, and so on); and (3) a public service organization to supply the volunteers who carry out the daily operations of the program.

Initial contact with the IHAF may come from any party interested in establishing a screening program. Written information and materials will be forwarded, and, when appropriate, a representative of the IHAF will be dispatched to assist in setting up a program (see Appendix 14–A).

The Professional

The professional serves a pivotal role within the IHAF organization, as well as constituting the primary link between the program and IHAF. The training and supervision of the volunteers, communication with hospital administration, as well as pediatric and nursing personnel, must all be coordinated by the professional. Interpretation of data and assurance of follow-up procedures are the exclusive domain of the professional. Initially, considerable time and effort are required to consolidate all components of the program. If such an individual is not readily available on staff, the hospital must make appropriate arrangements with a local audiologist or audiological service. Once the program is in place, the volunteers prepare risk registers, make appointments, carry out screening, and so on, thereby freeing the professional to conduct other business (see below).

Because some professionals have had limited experience with ABR technology or its application to the neonate, the IHAF has recently established a number of regional training centers. Appendix 14–B outlines the procedures used by Judith Marlowe, IHAF program director at Winter Park, Florida.

Volunteerism

In 1983, the IHAF received the President's Volunteer Action Award. This recognition rightfully belongs to the Chapters of the Telephone Pioneers of America, who have worked tirelessly over the years to make the hearing screening programs a success. In doing so, they have earned the admiration and respect of the professional community. Recently, the American Legion and International Lions have joined their ranks, and participation by other groups is encouraged. Currently, there are more than 1,000 volunteers involved in IHAF programs throughout the United States and Canada. The number of volunteers affiliated with a given program ranges from approximately 10 to 50, depending on the size of the nursery and its birth census.

Prior to actual screening of infants, the volunteers undergo extensive training. They are fully acquainted with hospital rules and protocol, as well as ABR recording techniques.

The Test Unit

The Synap I is a portable, user-friendly, microcomputer-based dedicated averaging device about the size of the proverbial "breadbox" (Fig. 14–1). It was designed for lay persons (volunteers) to operate with a minimum of instruction or experience.

By entering a simple code via the pressure-sensitive keypad, the volunteer can readily alter test parameters, such as the ear to be stimulated, intensity level, stimulus delivery rate, and so on. Feedback as to the status of the system is continuously presented through an 8-digit (LED) display window. A hard copy of the analog waveforms, as well as pertinent test information, is automatically printed following each run. The test results can optionally be stored on magnetic tape. The data collected with the Synap I are of the highest quality. Comparisons with expensive commercial averagers are most favorable (Fig. 14–2).

Because all software is contained on EPROMS (erasable programmable read only memory), modifications and upgrades are easily distributed and installed in units throughout the country. For complete details of the Synap I, refer to Salamy and Amochaev (1984), Salamy, Amochaev, and Sommerville (1983), and Salamy, Somerville, and Patterson (1982).

The Foundation supplies the Synap I, a preamplifier, a set of TDH-39 earphones, and a Users Guide to each new program. Several

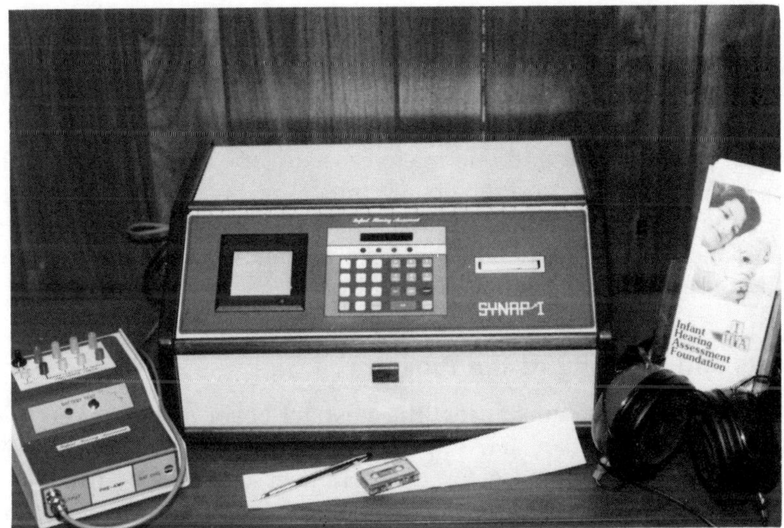

Figure 14–1. Synap I IHAF test unit with preamplifier (left) and the headphones (right).

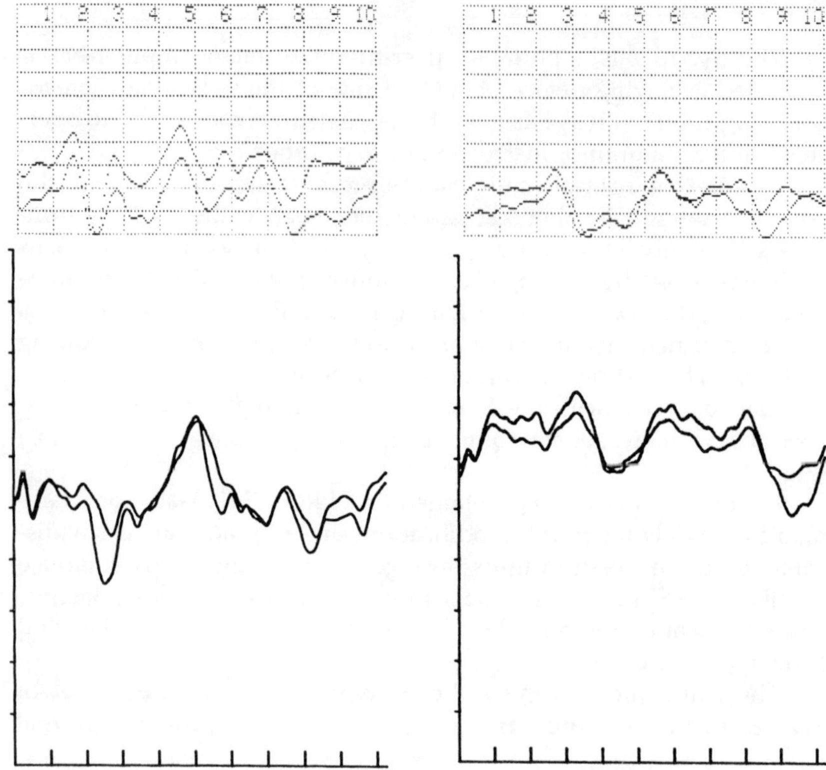

Figure 14–2. ABR's obtained from a young infant with the Synap I (upper tracings) and Nicolet Pathfinder (lower tracings). Note comparable resolution and replicability across units.

rolls of printer paper and one micro cassette tape are also furnished. The IHAP maintains and repairs all units at no cost to the participating program. Several field stations provide regional support. The Foundation retains ownership of the Synap I at all times. If a program terminates, the Synap I is returned.

Costs and Funding of the Program

Under most circumstances, the hospital bears no direct cost for the installation of an IHAF program. However, the hospital is required to provide space for the volunteer operations—usually a small room near the nursery, with telephone lines and general maintenance. The minimum amount of materials needed to conduct the ABR tests (e.g., electrodes, gel, cotton balls) as well as paper and cassette tapes for the Synap I unit are also supplied by the hospital.

Most often, all courtesies and privileges afforded to other volunteer groups in the hospital (e.g., parking, cafeteria passes) are also extended to IHAF volunteers. The professional's salary and percent effort is strictly between the hospital and the individual selected to oversee the program.

Funds for the placement of each successive program are derived primarily from four distinct sources: (1) corporate and personal donations, (2) grants, (3) revenues from ABR tests, and (4) fund raisers by the sponsoring organization. A continuous effort is made to obtain funds in the form of grants from other foundations, institutes, or large companies. The Foundation recommends that a fee determined exclusively by the hospital be levied for the ABR tests. Parents are never billed directly, and no one is denied the test for lack of coverage. The income actually collected from third party carriers (i.e., insurance companies, state agencies) is equally divided between the hospital and the Foundation. In this regard, it should be pointed out that a growing number of states are passing legislation mandating some form of infant hearing screening, particularly for intensive care nursery (ICN) survivors. Thus, some funds are being made available for ABR testing.

Clearly, one of the Foundation's principal means of support comes from fund raising projects undertaken by the volunteers in their home community. This may involve a golf or bowling tournament or a run or walk or may simply be a part of other ongoing activities from which some percentage of the proceeds are allocated to IHAF. Volunteer groups wishing to participate in a screening program must be willing to sponsor occasional fund raising drives.

Finally, mention should be made of contributions in the form of products, that is, electronic components, equipment, cassette tapes, or services and expertise offered ''at cost'' or free to the Foundation from corporations and companies of all sizes. For example, many of the computer chips used by the Synap I are donated by the Intel Corporation. Tymshare supplied computer lines and terminals. The royalties derived from a series of telephone decanters (historic models) distributed by Jim Beam Distilling Company provided a main source of funding for more than 4 years. Western Electric offered manufacturing skills, Braemar Computer Devices supplied the tape drives, and Hewlett-Packard donated test equipment. The dot matrix printers came from Gulton, the control panels (keyboard) from Molex, and 3M Company supplied the thermal paper, and Verbatim contributed some micro cassette tapes. A special debt of gratitude is owed to the retirees at the Western Electric Plant in Indianapolis, who assembled all existing Synap I units. Future models of the test set will be based on a commercial microcomputer.

MODEL PROGRAM: METHODIST HOSPITAL, INDIANAPOLIS, INDIANA

This program has been in operation since 1979 and was one of our first "high-risk" screening centers. It now serves as a model for both new and existing programs. The hospital has approximately 3500 births per year and a 20-bed ICN (Level III).

Initiation of the IHAF Program

Prior to the IHAF involvement, an informal attempt to screen newborns using the risk register and behavioral audiometry proved unsatisfactory. Once the IHAF came to the attention of the audiologist, negotiations between the Foundation, Telephone Pioneers, Hospital administration, and neonatology began. The program's organization and goals were explained by the audiologist to all parties in a series of meetings. To the audiologist, an IHAF program meant full-fledged screening of all high-risk infants, with only a relatively small increase in time required; to the hospital, it meant no monetary outlays, no expensive instrumentation, and no additional staffing; to the nursery personnel (pediatricians, neonatologists, nurses), it meant objective hearing screening for their clients.

To facilitate the start-up process, the Foundation provided a "working agreement" (Appendix 14–C), delineating the respective roles of each party. Once signed by all concerned, this served as the contractual basis for the program. Although not legally binding, the moral and ethical commitment is clear. In view of wide variations in hospital policy across the nation, this document basically represents a set of guidelines specifying the essential elements of a viable IHAF program.

Training of Volunteers

The training of the first group of volunteers required a considerable expenditure of time on the part of the audiologist. Subsequent training of new recruits is now carried out by experienced volunteers with the professional conducting occasional update and review sessions (e.g., quarterly).

To expedite the training sequence, the Foundation supplied a manual with information general enough for most hospital environments. Topics covered in the manual include hospital rules and regulations; key locations, such as the nursery, mothers' rooms, infants' charts; how to interview mothers; and how to handle infants. Volunteers were fully apprised of what was expected of them.

Once the volunteers felt comfortable with these tasks and the audiologist was satisfied with their level of performance, they were familiarized with anatomy and physiology of the auditory system and hearing disorders. At this time, they were introduced to ABR techniques. They were versed on the limits of the test and conditions that affect the results, that is, degree of maturity, baby's state (quiescent or active), electrical interference, artifacts, and so on. The importance of earphone position, electrode placement and impedance, as well as response reliability, were amply discussed. Extensive practice sessions were scheduled, with volunteers serving as subjects before screening babies (Table 14–1).

In addition to ABR testing, selected volunteers were trained to give brief presentations to the pre-natal classes and distribute developmental brochures. The volunteers also type and mail reports, prepare the data (ABR tracings) for the professional, and make appointments for follow-up evaluation. Once in place, the volunteers continue to run the program with the audiologist in a supervisory capacity.

At the onset, strenuous efforts were used to ensure support from the hospital staff (e.g., neonatology, pediatrics, nursing). Staff members were also encouraged to express appreciation to the volunteers.

A recurring concern pertains to the protection of confidentiality. At Methodist Hospital, initially, only a Pioneer who happened to be a nurse was permitted to examine the medical charts to make at-risk judgments. Generally speaking, if left up to the professional staff, completion of the risk register proves too tedious and time consuming and is subsequently neglected or abandoned. This is particularly true in a large ICN.

If confidentiality presents a major obstacle, the Foundation recommends that all ICN infants be tested, thereby circumventing the issue entirely. There is a growing recognition for the need to screen all ICN survivors, and this is becoming the standard practice in many hospitals. Of course, this would be totally untenable without a cadre of volunteers to do the work. An alternative is for a pediatrician or nurse to refer all infants with risk factors for ABR testing. The value of the risk register, particularly in the well-baby nursery or with infants receiving Level II care, cannot be minimized. Therefore, every attempt is made to include a risk register with the IHAF program. At Methodist Hospital, volunteers were initially allowed to interview mothers only to screen candidates. However, once their record of performance was established, they were approved to review charts and complete risk registers. The close supervision of the volunteers as well as their personal integrity eventually dispelled all concerns with regard to confidentiality. Following a 6-month trial period, the

Table 14–1. Summary of Data from Methodist Hospital's Infant Hearing Assessment Program

	NICU ABR		Follow-up ABR		Lost to Follow-Up	Confirmed Hearing Loss (Percentages based on total infants tested)				
Total	1090		168		53	66				
						Conductive	Sensorineural (3.85%)			
	Pass	Fail	Pass	Fail		Moderate Bilateral	Mild Bilateral	Moderate Bilateral	Severe Bilateral	Severe Unilateral
Number	869*	221	97	71†		24	6	20	12	4
%	79.7	20.2	57.7	42.2		2.2	0.6	1.8	1.1	0.4

* 2 infants with normal ABR responses in the NICU were identified with moderate to severe sensorineural hearing loss after 8 months of age.
† 5 infants who failed the retest subsequently died.

IHAF program was fully accepted at Methodist Hospital. Gerkin and Weyland (1985) also reported the successful utilization of the IHAF program in Indianapolis, Indiana, and Denver, Colorado.

Test Protocol

The test protocol used at Methodist Hospital, as well as other aspects of the program, have evolved over the years. In 1983, a conference was held in Vail, Colorado, for all IHAF program directors and affiliates. Its purpose was to share information and experiences, as well as to establish guidelines for new and existing programs. The attendees were representatives of a regional cross-section of IHAF facilities ranging from large urban centers to small rural and community hospitals. The group of approximately 25 professionals, including audiologists, pediatricians, physiologists, and psychologists was divided into several subcommittees to formulate general test procedures and pass-fail criteria. At a subsequent meeting in San Francisco, guidelines for follow-up were determined. The results of these two deliberations are presented in Appendix 14–D and 14–E. The guidelines are meant solely to provide a framework or model with the understanding that local contingencies must prevail. However, those willing to adhere to a uniform methodology can contribute and share information from an IHAF network now being created to establish a national data-pool.

Results

Following a protocol similar to that suggested in the IHAF guidelines, Methodist Hospital has successfully used volunteers to screen high-risk infants in the ICN. A carefully planned follow-up program at the hospital confirmed a significant number of infants with hearing loss. A summary of the program's results is presented in Table 14–1.

CONCLUSIONS

The model program described above attests to the strength of the IHAF organization. Interest and support for the IHAF continues to grow. As of this writing, there are 47 IHAF programs. Five of these are designated as research centers. In 1984, almost 1,000 volunteers logged more than 45,000 hours (estimate based on programs reporting) working on IHAF projects. Approximately 60,000 babies were born in IHAF hospitals, and 40,000 risk registers were completed. Of these, 8,000 babies were identified as at-risk, and 4,000 ABR tests were conducted. About 16.5 percent failed the initial screening. With thousands of infants receiving screening tests, there can be little doubt about the power and effectiveness of the IHAF system.

REFERENCES

Gerkin, K., and Weyland, C. (1985). Infant hearing assessment foundation programs. *Hearing Instruments, 36*(3), 22–24.

Salamy, A., and Amochaev, A. (1984). A practical approach to hearing of the newborn and at-risk infant. *Seminars in Hearing, 5,* 39–48.

Salamy, A., Amochaev, A., and Somerville, G. (1983). The IHAF screening device. *Hearing Instruments, 34,* 16–18.

Salamy, A., Somerville, G., and Patterson, D. (1982). The infant hearing assessment program. *Hearing Aid Journal, 35,* 10–13.

Appendix **14–A**
Regional IHAF Representatives

Alex Amochaev, Ph.D., Executive Director
Alan Salamy, Ph.D., Scientific Director
Galen E. Somerville, Engineer

National Headquarters: 4280 Hale Parkway, Denver, CO 80220
(303) 398-9036

East: Judith A. Marlowe, M.A., CCC, Director of Training and Programs, Winter Park Memorial Hospital, 200 North Lakemont Avenue, Winter Park, FL 32792, (305) 646-7000.

Mid West: Christina Weyland, M.A., CCC, Director, Infant Hearing Assessment Program, Methodist Hospital of Indiana, 1604 North Capitol Avenue, Indianapolis, IN 46202, (317) 929-3311.

Rocky Mountains: Katherine Pike Gerkin, M.A., CCC, Coordinator of Newborn Hearing Screening, University of Colorado Health Sciences Center, Audiology Division, 4200 East Ninth Avenue, Denver, CO 80262, (303) 394-7856.

West: Alan Salamy, Ph.D., Brain Behavior Research Center, Sonoma Development Center, University of California, Eldredge, CA 94531.

Appendix 14–B
Infant Hearing Assessment Foundation Training Program at Winter Park, Florida

DESCRIPTION

A 2-day program conducted at Winter Park Memorial Hospital for IHAF participating professionals and volunteer chairpersons. Using a demonstration-discussion-practicum format, the procedures necessary for conducting an IHAF program will be covered. These include infant history review, administration of evoked potential screening, record keeping, and volunteer training.

OBJECTIVES

The following instructional objectives will be met. Participants will demonstrate the ability to

1. Gown and scrub properly in accordance with hospital standards.
2. Identify the risk factors for hearing established by the Joint Committee (1983).
3. Review a hospital chart to locate information necessary to complete the IHAF Infant History Form.
4. Identify the location and function of the controls for the Synap unit.
5. Conduct self-test procedures for the pre-amp and main unit, including loop-around and RMS tests.
6. Apply electrodes in preparation for the test, including checks of electrode integrity, site preparation, use of the appropriate montage, and procedures for impedance measurement at electrode sites.
7. Follow the command sequence for administration of the ABR with the Synap, using the recommended protocol for intensity levels to be tested.
8. Apply criteria for determining when technically acceptable tracings have been obtained.
9. Interpret ABR tracings according to the recommended IHAF criteria for *screening,* as well as in follow-up (professional only).
10. Complete record keeping and a monthly report form.
11. Design a follow-up plan for repeat ABR and conventional audiometric assessment.
12. Plan for recruitment of additional volunteers, their on-site training, and methods for retaining their participation to enhance the longevity of the program.
13. Plan for community awareness campaigns to address the importance of early identification and the benefits of the IHAF program.

Appendix **14–C**
Memorandum of Agreement

AREAS OF RESPONSIBILITY

Hospital

A. Provide space convenient to the newborn nursery for testing and for general administration of the program with telephone access and furniture.
B. Work with volunteer group and audiologist to arrange test schedule.
C. Provide volunteers with standard facility identification, regular dining privileges (and rates), and parking privileges, and so on, similar to those afforded other hospital volunteers.
D. Provide that each volunteer is covered by sponsoring hospital's liability insurance policy.
E. Provide supplies to conduct ABR tests (e.g., electrodes, electrode gel, alcohol swabs, cotton balls, Q-tips, printer paper, cassette tapes).
F. Arrive at a cooperative financial plan in which:
    1. All at-risk infants will be tested, with consent of parents or physician, regardless of ability to pay.
    2. Assess a fee for ABR tests whereby parents are covered by third-party carriers (e.g., insurance, state agencies) or for each ''risk register'' completed.
    3. Share revenues collected with the Infant Hearing Assessment Foundation on a 50-50 basis.
G. Provide a billing mechanism, and forward a quarterly statement to the Foundation indicating the number of tests performed, amount billed, and amount collected.
H. Send quarterly payment directly to the Infant Hearing Assessment Foundation.
I. Obtain the services of an audiologist to direct the program. This individual will be knowledgable in ABR technology and experienced in infant recordings and interpretations. The audiologist's responsibilities will include
    1. Organize program.
    2. Train and supervise volunteers.
    3. Make at-risk determination.
    4. Ensure that all at-risk and referred infants are tested regardless of ability to pay, with concurrence of parents and physicians.
    5. Interpret test results.
    6. Implement follow-up procedures, and recommend appropriate referrals for treatment or remediation.
    7. Prepare ''monthly activity report'' for the Foundation.
J. Provide technical support to volunteer organization.
K. Help in the over-all training of the volunteers regarding hospital protocol.

Volunteer Organization

A. Assist in training volunteer staff.
B. Designate group leader who will
    1. Schedule daily coverage for the required hours of duty.
    2. Provide for back-up coverage in case of absence.
    3. Schedule initial and follow-up ABR tests as requested by audiologist and hospital staff.
    4. Coordinate volunteer activities with maternity, newborn nursery, and other hospital groups to ensure that the program's work is accomplished in a timely and efficient manner with a minimum of disturbance to established hospital routine.
    5. Schedule out-patient ABR tests as requested by attending pediatricians, audiologists, and parents.
C. Complete a risk register on each infant comprised of information obtained from
    1. Mother's hospital chart.
    2. Baby's hospital chart.
    3. Personal interview with parents (as necessary).
D. Give completed risk registers to audiologist for at-risk determination.
E. Perform ABR test on at-risk infants as directed, using SYNAP I Infant Screening Assessment Unit.
F. Prepare folder containing test result printouts for audiologists.
G. Perform outpatient and follow-up ABR tests as directed, and give results to audiologist.
H. Provide mother with folder listing the language acquisition indicators and encouraging her to follow her baby's progress.
I. Complete "Monthly Activity Report" and mail as prescribed. Audiologist will provide information on at-risk and hearing-impaired findings. Numbers of cases billed will agree with hospital and audiologist records.
J. Help to organize parent groups for education, mutual support, and encouragement.
K. Provide pamphlets telling about the program for new mothers and mothers-to-be at offices of obstetricians, pediatricians, family practitioners, ENT, and so on, in the area.
L. Explain program to service clubs, church groups, and so on.
M. Speak to parents attending obstetrical classes, prenatal tours, maternity teas, and so on.
N. Maintain health standards as prescribed by the hospital. Any required tests are provided by hospital at no charge to volunteer.
O. Maintain respect for total confidentiality of information that he or she has access to at all times, and do not disclose any information relating to infant tests or other knowledge obtained to anyone other than authorized staff members who have a need for the information.
P. Arrange for flexible duty hours to meet the needs of the program, determined jointly by hospital staff and volunteer group.
Q. Provide lab costs.

Infant Hearing Assessment Foundation

A. Provide SYNAP I assessment unit with actual ownership retained by the Infant Hearing Assessment Foundation.
B. Service and maintain SYNAP I through local affiliate and central support.
C. Provide materials, initial set of forms, training manual, testing equipment, and so on, associated with the program.
D. Provide Infant Hearing Assessment Foundation insignias to go on lab coats.

Other Guidelines

A. In the event that either the hospital or volunteers provide information for publication or respond to the media about the program at the hospital, proper credits should be given to all parties and to the Infant Hearing Assessment Foundation for their roles in providing this service. Volunteers, hospital, and hearing professionals should have the opportunity to review such material before it is released for publication or broadcast.
B. The Infant Hearing Assessment Program may be terminated by either the hospital, the sponsoring volunteer group, or by the Infant Hearing Assessment Foundation upon 30 days notice or upon a given length of time mutually agreed upon.

Appendix **14–D**
IHAF Vail Conference

PROTOCOL

1. Test all high-risk infants. All NICU, if possible. Use Joint Committee Criteria.
2. Bilateral Test, i.e., each ear tested separately.
3. Recommended montage: placement anywhere from vertex to hairline along midline to ipsilateral earlobe with contralateral earlobe as ground.
4. Check electrode impedance prior to first run for each ear.
5. Impedance values within 2000 ohms of each other at all sites and, when possible, under 10,000 ohms.
6. Use TDH-49 earphones.
7. 1200 clicks at 16 clicks per second. Run levels 2 and 3 or 4. If overlay is poor:
   a. Check earphone for presence of clicks.
   b. Check electrode:
      (1) Post position
      (2) Impedance
      (3) BER button
   c. Run level 0 control.
   d. Rerun test and continue.
8. Note infant state for each run.
9. Baby to be tested with head turned to side.
10. All electrodes the same; do not mix metals.
11. Follow-up of all high-risk infants is recommended.

PASS-FAIL CRITERIA

Pass—Presence of waves III or V at level 2 in both ears.

Retest—Any response other than clear pass to rule out technical errors.

> Two inconclusive screenings should constitute a referral for full audiological evaluation.

Optimally, initial screening is to be completed within 1 week of discharge.

Appendix **14–E**
IHAF San Francisco Conference

RECOMMENDATIONS FOR FOLLOW-UP

1. Infants who pass the initial ABR screening (acceptable tracings) should be followed by telephone interview with the parents at 4 months. A second telephone contact should be made at 8 months adjusted age. This is the final contact unless questionable hearing is reported. If any concerns about the baby's hearing are reported, a second ABR should be scheduled. If an infant fails this screening, the pediatrician should be notified and referrals should be made as below.

2. Infants who fail the initial ABR screening should be rescreened before leaving the hospital or returned within 2 weeks to rule out technical or transient problems. The pediatrician should also be alerted. If an unacceptable response is again observed, the infant should immediately be referred for behavioral screening and habilitation once the pediatrician is notified.

A protocol for the basic follow-up assessment was recommended in order to emphasize that the ABR alone must not be used to establish a diagnosis. In addition to a full latensity-intensity ABR, sound room testing should include noisemakers, warbled puretones, filtered tones, speech signals, startle responses by air and bone conduction, and impedance studies with acoustic reflexes. Otological examination and pediatric assessment for genetic and systemic factors are also recommended.

Author Index

A

Abrams, I. F., 36
Achor, L. J., 74
Ahlfors, K., 12, 39
Alberti, R. W., 89, 90, 93
Alford, C. A., 38, 39
Altman, M. M., 123, 238
Amlie, R. N., 69, 71, 74, 79
Amochaev, A., 104, 243
Amos, C. S., 39
Apgar, V., 33

B

Balkany, T. J., 4, 34, 43
Barrand, N., 124
Battaglia, F. C., 35
Beck, T., 124
Beggs, F., 134
Behrman, R. E., 33, 34, 35
Berenberg, W., 39
Bergstrom, L., 6, 8, 37, 107, 123, 238
Berlow, S. J., 35
Berman, S. A., 4, 34, 43
Black, F. O., 37
Borkowska-Gaertig, D., 9

Branigan, P. W., 37
Bronshvag, M., 80
Brown, W. N., 37
Buda, F. B., 69
Budetti, P., 124
Bull, D., 68
Brukhard, R., 74, 76, 79, 80, 83
Burney, P., 48

C

Caldarelli, D. D., 35
Campbell, A. M. G., 36
Campbell, K. B., 73, 82
Cann, J., 82
Carrel, R. E., 70
Cevette, M. S., 74, 93, 104
Chandler, D., 47, 48
Chaplin, E. R., 71
Chasin, J., 47, 48
Chomsky, N., 6
Cinnamond, M. J., 37
Clark, B. R., 43
Clark, L. F., 82
Clark, S., 101, 104
Clark, T., 123
Clark, T. C., 230
Clements, P. A. R., 76

Clifton, F., 36
Clinton-Brown, K., 93
Coats, A. C., 83
Coen, R. W., 71
Cone, B. K., 74, 184
Conry, R. F., 43
Corbin, H., 89, 90, 93
Corfits, J. L., 76, 78, 80, 83
Cox, L. C., 70, 71, 74, 76, 78, 93, 104
Crump, B., 48
Cunningham, G. C., 12, 32

D

D'Souza, S. W., 34
Dahle, A. J., 39
Dale, R., 47, 48
Davey, P. R., 43
Davis, H., 70, 92, 93, 104, 124
Davis, J. M., 6, 7
Delk, M. T., 3, 4
Dennis, J. M., 93
Desmont, G., 36
Despland, P., 74, 76, 78, 80, 104
Dodge, P. R., 35
Doehring, D. G., 11
Donohue, J. F., 37
Downs, D. W., 9, 70, 124
Downs, M. P., 6, 8, 10, 11, 21, 31, 37, 40, 47, 48, 69, 107, 123, 184, 229, 238
Doyle, D. J., 84
Doyle, W. J., 74, 76
Drillen, C. M., 43
Durieux-Smith, A., 64, 65, 69, 74, 76, 79, 80, 81, 93, 103, 104

E

Edwards, C. G., 64, 65, 69, 74, 76, 79, 80, 81, 103
Eggermont, J. J., 74
Ehrlich, C. H., 123
Eichwald, J., 130, 224
Elberling, C., 69
Elliott, S., 76
Ermocilla, R., 39
Etienne, J. E., 123

F

Feigin, R. D., 35
Feinmesser, M., 9, 12, 32, 47, 48, 69, 123, 184, 238
Felix, J. K., 29, 93
Fenn, B. C., 80
Finitzo-Hieber, T., 35, 74, 93
Fitch, J. L., 123
Fitzhardinge, P. M., 89
FitzZaland, R. E., 130
Fleming, W. L., 37
Frankenburg, W., 8, 9
Fraser, G. R., 41
Fredericks, W. R., 41
Fria, T. J., 74, 76, 92, 93, 158
Froding, C. A., 10

G

Gafni, M., 79
Galambos, C., 47, 62, 64, 69
Galambos, R., 47, 62, 64, 69, 70, 71, 73, 74, 76, 78, 80, 81, 91, 93, 100, 104, 124
Gaylor, D. W., 130, 224, 237
Gerber, S. E., 48, 69, 124
Gerkin, K. P., 8, 32, 39, 86, 249
Giebink, G. S., 4
Goldstein, P. J., 29, 93
Goldstein, R., 11
Gollegly, K. M., 167
Goodman, T. T., 64, 65, 103
Gorga, M. P., 6, 7
Gorlin, R. J., 38
Green, H. G., 130, 224, 237
Greenstein, B. B., 5, 8
Greenstein, J. M., 5, 8
Gross, S., 79
Guinagh, B. J., 7, 9

H

Hack, M., 70, 71, 76, 93, 104
Hankla, J., 129
Hanshaw, J. B., 38
Hanson, V., 41
Harford, E. R., 4
Harris, I., 41

Harris, K. C., 29, 93
Harris, S., 12, 39
Harsch, G. G., 35
Hecox, K., 69, 73, 74, 76, 78, 79,
        80, 83
Heiner, L., 124
Hemenway, W. G., 6, 8, 11, 47,
        107, 123, 238
Henther, M., 123
Hicks, G. E., 70, 71, 74, 91, 93,
        104, 124
Hirsch, A., 124
Hoffman, H. E., 39
Holson, J. F., 130, 224, 237
Hyde, M. L., 78, 84, 89, 90, 91,
        93, 104
Hyman, C. B., 41

I

Ivarsson, S., 12, 39

J

Jabaley, T. J., 102, 160
Jacobson, J. T., 69, 74, 76, 78, 79,
        80, 92, 93, 104
Jaffe, B. F., 40
James, L., 33
Jauhiainen, T., 123, 124, 239
Jester, R. E., 7, 9
Jewett, D. L., 73
Johansson, R., 123, 124, 239
Johnson, M. J., 74, 76, 78, 79, 80
Jones, F. R., 47, 49, 51, 52, 62, 184
Joint Committee on Infant hearing,
        69, 101, 160, 176, 239

K

Kankkunen, A., 35, 124
Karmody, C. S., 37
Katz, S., 34, 35, 37
Kaufman, L., 77
Kavesch, D. A., 39
Keaster, V., 41
Keith, R. W., 48
Kerley, S. M., 124
Kerr, A., 37

Kerrick, G. M., 39
Keyserling, H. L., 39
Kiang, N., 82
Kileny, P., 93, 104
Kimball, B. D., 123
Klein, J. O., 4, 35
Klein, N., 38
Knott, J., 82
Konigsmark, B. W., 38
Koops, B. L., 35
Kraus, N., 64, 93, 101, 104
Krugman, S., 34, 35, 37
Krumholz, A., 29, 93
Kuyper, P., 102

L

Le, C.T., 4
Lenneberg, E. H., 6, 123
Lernmark, B., 12, 39
Levi, H., 69, 123, 238
Levine, R. L., 41
Ling, A. H., 11
Ling, D., 11
Livan, M., 43
Livingston, M. M., 39
Loyd, D., 129
Luterman, D. M., 47, 48

M

MacMurray, B., 64, 65, 69, 74, 76,
        79, 80, 81, 103
Mageroy, K., 43
Magian, V.deC., 14
Mahoney, T., 124, 130, 139, 224,
        230
Maisels, M. J., 41
Marcellino, G. R., 63
Marcy, S. M., 35
Marshall, R. E., 70, 92, 104, 124
Martin, J. L., 83
Martin, W. H., 69, 71, 74, 79
Matz, G. J., 35
Mauldin, L., 48
McCaffee, M. A., 93
McCartney, E., 34
McClelland, R., 76
McCollister, F. P., 39

McConville, K., 5, 8
McCracken, G. H., 93
McCrae, M. Q., 108
McCrea, R., 76
McCulloch, B. J., 12, 32
McDermott, J. C., 4
McDonald, A., 4, 33, 43
McFarland, W. H., 47, 49, 51, 52,
    62, 69, 184
McKay, J. R., 33, 34, 35
McKean, C. M., 69, 76, 79, 80, 81
McManus, P., 124
Mencher, G. T., 12, 32, 69, 104,
    124, 125, 171, 184, 223
Mendelson, T., 71, 80
Metz, D. A., 70, 71, 76, 93, 104
Meyer, D. H., 35, 124
Miller, K., 63, 64, 103
Mohindra, O. D., 39
Mohr, J., 43
Mokotoff, B., 69
Moneka, W. J., 167
Morehouse, C. R., 69, 74, 76, 78,
    79, 80, 92, 93
Moroso, M., 90, 93
Murnane, O., 93, 104
Myers, G. J., 38, 39

N

Nahmias, A. J., 36, 39
Nankervis, G., 39
Nelson, C. J., 130, 224, 237
Nolan, M., 34
North, F. A., 9
Northern, J. L., 9, 11, 21, 39, 40,
    47, 48, 69, 123, 184, 229
Novotny, G. M., 76

O

Ozdamar, O., 64, 93

P

Paparella, M. M., 4, 35
Parrott, V., 104
Parving, A., 69
Pass, R. F., 38, 39
Paton, J., 64, 93
Patterson, D., 243
Pauwels, H. P., 76

Perez-Abalo, M., 91
Pettett, C., 80
Phon, G. L., 70, 92, 93, 104
Picton, T. W., 64, 65, 69, 73, 74,
    76, 79, 80, 81, 82, 91, 103
Pumper, R. W., 38

R

Rabak, L. P., 65
Rapin, I., 7
Rapoport, S. I., 41
Reed, D., 91
Reichert, T. J., 70, 92, 93, 104, 124
Reis, P., 6
Remein, Q. R., 21, 99
Remington, J. S., 35, 36
Reynolds, D. W., 39
Richards, I. D. G., 31
Riko, K., 89, 90, 93
Roberts, C. J., 31
Roberts, J. L., 70, 92, 93, 104
Robinson, M. J., 79
Rodman, S. M., 39
Rola-Janicki, A., 9
Romano, M. N., 73
Rosenthall, V., 35
Rosner, B. A., 4
Rousseeuw, P. J., 76
Ruben, R. J., 7, 48
Russ, F. W., 49
Rzedowskaz, 9

S

Salamy, A., 69, 71, 74, 76, 78, 79,
    80, 81, 93, 104, 243
Salmivalli, A., 123, 124, 239
Salomon, G., 69
Sanders, M. A., 104
Sanders, R., 93
Sanders, S., 69, 71, 74, 79
Sando, I., 38
Saxon, S. S., 39
Schein, J. D., 3, 4
Schneider, B. A., 68
Schuknecht, H. F., 37
Schulman-Galambos, C., 69, 70,
    78, 81, 93, 100
Schweinhart, L. J., 8
Sedgwick, R., 41
Seitz, M. R., 104

Shannon, D. A., 29, 93
Shapiro, E., 123
Sharbrough, F. W., 79, 80, 83
Shaw, C. P., 47, 48
Sheldon, R., 93
Shepard, N. T., 6, 7
Simmons, F. B., 34, 41, 47, 49, 51,
    52, 62, 63, 64, 69, 100, 103,
    124, 184
Simmons, M. A., 4, 43
Smith, A., 91
Smyth, G. D., 37
Sobieszanska-Radoszewska, L., 9
Sohmer, H., 79
Sommerville, G., 243
Sprinkle, P. M., 39
Stagno, S., 38, 39
Stapells, D. R., 73, 83, 91
Starr, A., 69, 71, 74, 79
Stein, L. K., 64, 93, 101, 102, 104,
    160
Stelmachowitz, P. G., 6, 7
Stensland-Junker, K., 9
Sterritt, G. M., 10, 31
Stewart, J., 124
Stick, S. L., 12
Stockard, J. E., 71, 74, 76, 78, 79,
    80, 83
Stockard, J. J., 71, 74, 76, 78, 79,
    80, 83
Strome, M., 37
Stubbs, K. G., 39
Sturtevant, E. M., 70, 92, 93, 104
Suguira, S., 35
Suonpaa, J., 123, 124, 239
Svanberg, L., 12, 39

T

Tait, C., 11
Taylor, I. G., 34
Teele, D. W., 4
Tell, L., 9, 12, 32, 123, 184, 238
Thomas, E., 82
Thompson, G., 69

Thorner, R. M., 21, 99
Tooley, W. H., 71
Toubas, P., 93
Trehub, S. E., 68

U

Urbanska, I., 9
U.S. Department of Health and
    Human Services, 107

V

Vaughn, V. C., 33, 34, 35
Veltry, R. W., 39
Vernon, J., 38
Vernon, M., 35
Vogeleer, M., 76

W

Watanabe, T., 82
Watkins, S., 230
Weber, H., 12, 133
Webster, D. B., 7
Webster, M., 7
Wedenberg, E., 10
Weikart, D. P., 8
Weizman, Z., 79
Weller, T. H., 38
Westmoreland, B. F., 76, 78, 80, 83
Weyland, C., 249
Williams, T. F., 123
Williston, J. S., 73
Wilson, M. J., 70, 71, 74, 91, 93,
    104, 124
Wilson, W. R., 39, 69
Wolfe, V., 124
Wood, R. P., 38
Wright, A. R., 41
Wright, L. B., 65
Wursten, H., 41

Y

Yamashiroya, H. M., 38

Subject Index

A

Academy of Pediatrics, 4
Acoustic impedance measurements, 48
Acute suppurative otitis media, 4, 34
Administrative staff, role in screening, 110
Alaska, large-scale screening program attempt, 136
address, 139
American Speech and Hearing Association, 11
Apgar score, 33, 34, 128, 231, 237
Arizona, state sponsored screening program, 136
address, 139
Arkansas, state-wide screening program, 134
address, 139
Asphyxia, as risk factor, 32–33, 125
hearing loss result, 34
At-risk register, well-baby nursery, 100–101
Audiologist, role in screening, 108
Auditory brainstem response, 8, 10, 11, 13
absolute-relative latencies, 74
click-generated, 78
drawbacks, 88–89
historical development, 68–69
interwave interval measurement, 73

maturational trends, 74–77, 75, 77
response features, 71
screening tool, 29, 48, 59, 64, 247
use by Children's Hospital, Oakland, California, 146
use by Children's Hospital, Pittsburgh, Pennsylvania, 157–158, 161
use by Prentice Women's Hospital and Maternity Center, Chicago, Illinois, 173–174, 178
use by Reading Hospital and Medical Center, Reading, Pennsylvania, 183–184, 187–188
yield, 92–93
Auditory screening of neonates, 47–48
behavioral (motor) responses, 48
high-risk register, 48
psysiological, 48
Auropalpebral response (APR), 10–11

B

Bacterial meningitis, 34–35, 125
hearing loss result, 35
Band-pass EEG filter, 83–84
Behavioral observation audiometry, 67–68

Behavioral screening, 171–712
Birth certificate, as screening
        device, 224
    computerized search, 231–239
    risk criteria analysis, *232, 233,
        234, 235*
    Utah certificate, *226*
Birmingham, Alabama, speech-
        hearing conference, 126
Bone-conduction testing, 92
Brain plasticity, 6–7
British Columbia, regional screen-
        ing program, 130–131
    address, 139

C

California, state mandated screen
        ing program, 135
    address, 139
Center for Children's Communica-
        tion Disotders, 146
    ABR use, 146–147
    cost effectiveness, 151
    Crib-o-gram use, 146–147
    flow chart, *148*
    neonatal follow-up program,
        149, 152
    screening failure incidence, *150*
    volunteer program, 147
Children's Hospital, Oakland,
        California, 145–146. See
        also *Center for Children's
        Communication Disorders.*
Children's Hospital, Pittsburgh,
        Pennsylvania, 157
    program development, 157–160
        cost determination, 158
        follow-up protocol, *162*
        high risk register, 161
        logistics, 160
        normative data collection, 159
        parents' information, 160
        primary care physicians, 159–
            169
        results, 163
        test protocol, 160–163
Chronological program flowchart,
        225
Click stimulus, 71, 77–78, *79*, 91–
        92, 161

parameters, 77–84
    band-pass filtering, 83–84
    electrode placement, 83
    initial fail rate, 103
    intensity, 78–80
    polarity, 82–83
    rate, 80–82
Cochlear pathology, 72–73
Colorado, state sponsored screen-
        ing program, 133
    address, 139
Computerized birth certificate
        search, 231–236
Conference on Newborn Hearing
        Screening, 145–146
Congenital infections, 35–39, 125
Craniofacial anomalies, 39–40, 125
    hearing loss result, 40
Crib-o-gram, 11, 49–65, 69, 145–
        146
    algorithm development, 53–56
    equipment, 49
    interstimulus level, 62–63, *64*
    microprocessor version, 56–59
    scoring, 49–51
    screening accuracy, 51, 103
    time windows, *50*
    use by the Center for Children's
        Communication Disorders,
        146–147
    volunteer program, 147
    use by Reading Hospital and
        Medical Center, Reading,
        Pennsylvania, 183–184
        186–187
    validation study, 59–62, 64–65
Cytomegalovirus (CMV), 12, 38–
        39, 125
    hearing loss result, 39

D

Deaf manpower earnings, 4–5
Decision matrix, 22–23, *23, 26*
Diagnosis-screening differentia-
        tion, 21–22
Differential preamplifier role, 83
Dominant inheritance, 41–42

E

Early hearing assessment programs, general goals, 85
program design, 85
selection procedures, 85–87
test methods, 90–92
test timing, 88–89
test validity, 87
Early home language stimulation
programs, 7–9
Electrocochleography, 48
Electroencephalographic activity,
83
Electrode placement, 83

F

Family history, deafness result, 41–
43, 124–125
Florida, state mandated screening
program, 132
address, 139
Follow-up testing, 117

G

Gallaudet College survey, 5–6
Georgia, state sponsored screening
program, 129
address, 140
Governmental agencies involvement, mass newborn high-
risk hearing screening,
125–126

H

Hearing impaired language skills,
developmental patterns, 5–
6
Hearing impairment, demographic
figures, 3–4
Hearing loss explanation form, 154
Hearing screening results, recording form, 153
Herpes simplex virus, 39, 125
hearing loss result, 39
High-risk register, 31–33, 48, 101,
113–114, 123, 124, 160, *161*,
183–184, 186, 238–239

Hospital-based hearing screening
program, 107–108, 124
administrative staff-personnel
role, 110
audiologist's role, 108
cost-reimbursement, 118
follow-up, 117
implementation, 118–119
neonatologist's role, 109
nursing staff, 109–110
otolaryngologist's role, 109
record keeping, 117–118
screening process, 111–113
Hyperbilirubinemia, 12, 18, 40–41,
125, 167
hearing loss result, 41
suggested exchange transfusion
levels, 42
Hypoxia, 12, 125

I

IHAF San Francisco Conference,
257
IHAF Vail Conference, 256
Infant Hearing Assessment Foundation, 241
model program, 246–247
data summary, *248*
memorandum of agreement,
253–255
regional representatives, 251
San Francisco Conference, 257
test protocol, 249
Vail Conference, 256
volunteer training, 246–247
Winter Park Memorial Hospital, Florida, training program, 252
program components, 241–242
professional role, 242
program funding, 244–245
Synap I test unit, 243–244
volunteerism, 242
Intensive care nursery, 145, 247–
248
International Conference on Early
Diagnosis of Hearing Loss,
69
Interwave interval, 72–73

Iowa public schools, hearing
impaired children report, 6,
7, 7

J

Joint Committee on Infant Hearing, 11
categories of risk selection, 12
high-risk register, 32–33, 101,
113–114, 123, 128, 160, 171,
184, 223, 226
position statement, 17–19, 69,
85, 86, 124–125

L

Language, as innate function, 6–7
Language learning, early implementation importance, 7–8
Large-scale screening programs,
123–127, 139–140
birth certificate data use, 127–129
hospital questionnaire use, 130–
136
Letter to parents, 181
Lexington School for the Deaf, 8
Low birthweight, hearing loss risk,
43, 125
otitis media relationship, 43

M

Magee Women's Hospital, 157, 160
Massachusetts, state mandated
screening program, 131
address, 140
Methodist Hospital, Indianapolis,
Indiana, 246
IHAF model program, 246–249
data summary, *248*
test protocol, 249
volunteer training, 246–247
Middle ear effusion, 4
Mothers' instructional pamphlet,
198–206

N

Nager's syndrome, 149
National Meeting of Directors of
Speech and Hearing Pro-
grams in State Health and
Welfare Agencies, 125–126
Neonatal hearing loss, estimates of
incidence, 47
Neonatal screening alternatives, 8–
9
Neonatologist, role in screening,
109
New Jersey, state mandated
screening program, 131–132
address, 140
Nicolet Pathfinder, 244
Northwestern Perinatal Center. See
*Prentice Women's Hospital
and Maternity Center*
Nova Scotia, comprehensive
screening program, 134
address, 140
Nova Scotia Conference, 124–125,
136, 171, 223
Nurses' instructional pamphlet,
207–210
Nursing staff, role in screening,
109–110

O

Ohio, state sponsored screening
program, 135
address, 140
Oklahoma, state sponsored
screening program, 132–133
address, 140
Otolaryngologist, role in screening, 109

P

Parent-Infant Program, Utah, 230
Parent information, hearing
screening program, 113
Pediatrician, role in screening, 108
Perinatal infections. See *Congenital
infections.*
Physician letter, screening failure
report, 155
Polarity measurement, 82–83
Prentice Women's Hospital and
Maternity Center, Chicago,
Illinois, 165
audiology program organization,
166–167, *168, 169, 170,*
170–171

administration-cost considerations, 175
follow-up method, 175–176
habilitation, 176–177
nursery screening results, 177–
179, *178*
results reporting, 174–175
risk factors criteria, 166–167
screening protocol, 172–177
pass criteria, 173
response scale, 172
stimuli,172
Prevalence of impairment influence, in testing, 25–26
Public health screening, criteria, 9–
10

R

Random neonatal response rate,
51
Reading Hospital and Medical
Center, Reading, Pennsyl-
vania, 183
hearing screening program
development, 183–184
administrative considerations,
189
auditory brainstem response
screening, 187
crib-o-gram screening, 186
high-risk register, 186
initial and current high-risk
registers, *185*
letters to parents, 214, 221
letters to pediatricians, 211–
213, 215–219
medical clearance form, 220
mothers' pamphlet, 198–206
nurses' instructional pamphlet, 207–210
one year questionnaire, 188–
189, 222
results reporting, 189–192
data summary, *190, 192*
screening report form, 195–197
screening protocol, 184–186
flow chart, *185*
seven month audiological
testing, 188
Recessive inheritance, 42

Rubella, 12, 37–38, 125
hearing loss result, 38

S

Screening, definition, 9–10, 12–13
Screening feasibility study, 100–
101
Screening follow-up, 99–100, *104*
Screening level selection justification, 102–103
Screening method selection, 112–
113
target population, 112
Screening procedure checklist, 114
Screening programs, interprofessional collaboration, 110–
112
basic concepts, 110–112
Screening results, breakdown, 28
Sensitivity, in screening tests, 10,
11, 22
Specificity, in screening tests, 10,
11, 22
Stanford Achievement Test, paragraph meaning subtests
scores, *6*
Stanford University medical Center, Crib-o-gram study, 51,
53
State mandated screening programs, *127*, 139–140
Stimulus attenuation, 78–79
Stimulus repetition rate change,
80–83, *82*
Stimulus response latency interval,
51
Synap I, 243–244, *244*
model program, 246–249
Syphilis, 36–37, 125
hearing loss result, 37

T

Telephone Pioneers of America,
241, 242
Tennessee, state sponsored screening program, 129
address, 140
Test administration, 115–116
results-reports, 116

Tests, operating characteristics, 22–
23, 90–93
  cutoff score importance, 23–24,
    24
  over-referral rate, 25–26, 27
  percent sensitivity, 22
Tonepip ABR recording, 84
TORCH complex, 35–36, 166
Toxoplasmosis, 36, 125
  hearing loss result, 36

U

United States Department of
    Health and Human Serv-
    ices, 126
Utah Department of Health,
    Bureau of Communicative
    Disorders, 223–224
  computerized mass newborn
    screening, 223–224, 236–239
  program flow chart, 225
  program procedures, 224–231
    audiology center screening,
      228
    birth certificate use, 224–226,
      226
    diagnostic testing, 230
    itinerant clinic screening, 229–
      230
  parental notification, 227
  parental response card, 228
  referral and follow-up, 230–231
  risk criteria analysis, 232, 233,
    234, 235
Utah, state sponsored screening
    program, 127–128
  program outline, 128
  address, 140

V

Visual reinforcement audiometry, 68

W

Wave latency prolongation, 78–80
  age differences, 79, 80
Well-baby public health clinics, as
    neonatal screening alterna-
    tives, 9
Winter Park Memorial Hospital,
    Florida, 252
Wisconsin, state sponsored screen-
    ing program, 135
  address, 140

X

X-linked inheritance, 42–43